Praise for *She Rides*

"We all embark on journeys of discovery borhood or faraway lands, but few of us take on the rigors that Alenka Vrecek does in *She Rides*. The psychological and emotional challenges of this solo-cycling marathon from Lake Tahoe to southern Baja are as daunting as the physical ones, but she navigates them all, emerging from the experience having found what she was seeking: her place in the world."

—Larry Habegger, executive editor of Travelers' Tales Books

"*She Rides* is heartfelt and riveting from the opening lines. So much more than a grueling bicycle adventure; Vrecek openly shares her feelings of longing for her home country, the fallout from the dissolution of her first marriage, and the prospect that she might not recover from cancer. Ultimately, through courage, fortitude, and sheer badass strength, she makes the most important discovery of all: that she can unflinchingly face any challenge and confront every obstacle head-on, and that she's just fine being who she is."

—Michael Shapiro, author of *A Sense of Place*

"In *She Rides*, Alenka Vrecek finds inner strength and a community that crosses both borders and boundaries as she travels by mountain bike alone on backroads from Lake Tahoe, California, to La Ventana, Baja. Her exciting story will be inspirational—and maybe even a comfort—to women across the globe."

—Laura Read, journalist, photographer, and editor

"*She Rides* is a tale of the spunk, perseverance, and desire it took for Alenka to not only finish the ride but always live life to the fullest. It's also funny and humble, and a touching tribute to the human spirit."

—Tim Hauserman, author of *Going It Alone:*
Ramblings and Reflections from the Trail

SHE
RIDES

SHE
RIDES

Chasing Dreams Across California and Mexico

Alenka Vrecek

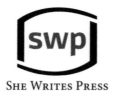

SHE WRITES PRESS

Published 2023
Printed in the United States of America
Print ISBN: 978-1-64742-456-5
E-ISBN: 978-1-64742-457-2
Library of Congress Control Number: 2022919269

For information, address:
She Writes Press
1569 Solano Ave #546
Berkeley, CA 94707

Interior Design by Kiran Spees

She Writes Press is a division of SparkPoint Studio, LLC.

All company and/or product names may be trade names, logos, trademarks, and/or registered trademarks and are the property of their respective owners.

Names and identifying characteristics have been changed to protect the privacy of certain individuals.

*For my father and mother who have always been
my guiding lights,*

*For my children, Mateja, Jana, and Tilen,
for whom my love knows no boundaries.*

*For my husband, Jim, who is strong enough to
love me for who I am.*

In memory of Rosalva and Omar.

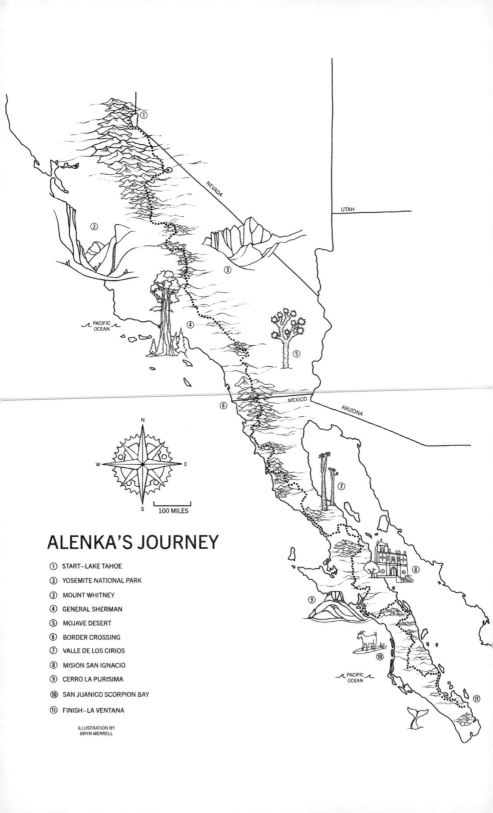

ALENKA'S JOURNEY

① START—LAKE TAHOE
② YOSEMITE NATIONAL PARK
③ MOUNT WHITNEY
④ GENERAL SHERMAN
⑤ MOJAVE DESERT
⑥ BORDER CROSSING
⑦ VALLE DE LOS CIRIOS
⑧ MISIÓN SAN IGNACIO
⑨ CERRO LA PURISIMA
⑩ SAN JUANICO SCORPION BAY
⑪ FINISH—LA VENTANA

ILLUSTRATION BY
BRYN MERRELL

Prologue

The sound of the groan surprises me. It is otherworldly. Barely human. Before I realize it's mine, sharp pain rushes through my right leg and arm. It feels as if a spoke from the wheel pierced my skin. I control my breathing: slow, shallow, quiet breaths, trying not to disturb the silence around me. As my gasps abate, I begin to take stock of my situation, slowly scanning my body from head to toe.

I am lying on my back, my head pointing downhill on a steep and rocky slope, wedged between two boulders. Jagged rocks jab my back and legs like a bed of nails. A small cactus pokes me in the ribs. The Beast, my sixty-five-pound mountain bike, lies awkwardly on top of me, pressing camping gear and supplies into my limbs and gut.

I can't move. I am too exhausted to do anything but watch the clouds as they roll across the hot, bright Mexican sky.

Is this it? Has death come for me? Here? Now? In the middle of this glorious day? All I see is white light. My feet and my hands prickle. Panic wells up. Am I dying? I want to pray to God to get me out of this mess, but I don't really know how. Growing up, I learned God, religion, and church were opiates for the masses. Yet, I've always prayed in my most desperate moments. I envied my two devout grandmothers for the comfort they found in God, and I liked going to sit in a quiet, cool, dark church with them, pretending to pray. So now I pray because I am desperate. Give me the strength, give me the will to move my body. I need to get back to my kids! I made a vow to them I'd never leave them. I must go back to Jim, my darling, my husband. I am overwhelmed by the feeling of guilt. Jim didn't want me to go on this adventure, and now he is going to be so mad at me if I die here.

I try to raise my head but can't.

I close my eyes again and start laughing, but the tears run into my ears.

"You goddamn idiot," I murmur. "You went on this trip to live, not to die!" I wiggle my toes. I wiggle my fingers. I squeeze my butt cheeks. Strange energy surges through me.

I breathe hot air and go over the crash in my head: my front wheel catching a sharp rock, shooting my bike hard to the right where it slides off the trail down a steep embankment. Quickly gaining speed as I fruitlessly pumped the brakes, I avoided two deadly boulders before bouncing off a third, the granite smoothed by centuries of erosion. It flipped me and my bike into the air, sending out a plume of camping gear, water bottles, and food, before catapulting The Beast and me to our awkward resting place.

I close my eyes again, and I realize that it's the fiftieth day since I left Lake Tahoe. Right now, home feels impossibly far away. My head starts spinning again, as if I am suddenly falling into the abyss. Haven't I been through enough in my life? Why did I go on this crazy bike trip all by myself? To tempt my fate? At fifty-four, I shouldn't have to do that. I shake my head and open my eyes. The hot desert sun blinds me, and I feel it on every inch of my body. Suddenly I realize how thirsty I am.

"Take me home," I whimper to the travel gods.

But where is that? I'm still not sure.

What I do know is that I'm hours away from help. I'm running low on water, and my emaciated, hundred-pound body is an easy snack for a predator, despite the fact there's no longer much meat on it.

You need to keep going, says a voice out of nowhere.

I tell the voice, *Go to hell!* It just laughs empathetically.

This makes me furious.

Inch by inch, I push off the bike and crawl from underneath it, moaning with pain while taking deep breaths in between. Finally, I am free of the burden of The Beast. I'm lying on my back, watching the clouds changing shapes, and in those shapes, I begin to see the antidote to death. I turn slowly from my back to my knees.

Okay, God, and the ancient spirits who roamed here before me. I am humble but not yet broken.

Now get me the hell out of here!

For once in my life, let me finish what I started. Don't let me fail. I beg of you. Let me climb this impossible mountain so I can go on living with the people I love.

It takes a tremendous effort to drag The Beast back onto the trail. Gear bags and water holders hang loosely. But I do it, if only to get away from the sanctimonious imaginary being giving me the world's worst pep talk. I begin picking up my scattered gear from the path of destruction. I lift my helmet and hold it in my hands, promising I'll keep it on my head at all times. I limp along for a while and then get back on the bike to slowly push my way to the top of the climb.

Time feels like it's running out, but I am not going to quit. Not yet.

I planned this trip for years, if only initially in my mind. At home in Lake Tahoe, my bookshelf is lined with stories written by climbers and explorers of exotic places and new frontiers. They circumnavigated the globe in sailboats, on foot, and by bike. I've always dreamed of scaling big mountains like Everest, crossing oceans on a windsurfer, sailing a boat solo around the world. But they were just someone else's dreams, struggles, and triumphs, distracting me from reality and the immediacy of everyday life, raising three kids. Someday, maybe someday, I told myself, I'll go and have my own adventure.

Years passed. The weight of it all began to suffocate me. I prayed to higher powers to take over every damn time that heavy black boot began pressing down on my chest, threatening to squeeze the last bit of air out of my lungs. I needed to get away so I could learn how to breathe again. This trip was supposed to be an emotional and physical pilgrimage. I wanted to see what I was still capable of. I needed to show myself and others that dying was not yet on my list of things to do. I left my home because I wanted to find, once and for all, the true meaning of life. My life.

This is no easy task for an immigrant who spent her entire adult life living in the space between nations and cultures. I have always felt a vague sense of exile from the place where I was born. I loved my native land of Slovenia deeply, but I also had a feverish urge to travel and explore unfamiliar places. While I own houses in Tahoe and Southern Baja, I have been in a perpetual search of a home, not just a place but a sense of belonging. I hoped I could connect all the dots of my life by riding door to door.

So now I'm here, in the rugged Sierra de la Giganta Mountains of the Baja California peninsula, where the temperature is already well over a hundred degrees. I've covered more than two thousand miles since I left Tahoe, riding along the spine of the Sierra Nevada, crossing the Mojave Desert before climbing back up to the San Gabriel Mountain Range. I climbed and descended the San Bernardino and

San Jacinto Mountains and, just before crossing the Mexican border, did the same in the Cuyamaca and Laguna Mountains.

All those miles turned my body into one giant saddle sore. My destination is the Bay of La Ventana, on the Sea of Cortez near the southern end of Baja, where my family has owned a small palapa for decades.

On a bike, one is always moving forward. Only by doing that did I think I would be able to feel alive again. I only needed to prove myself to myself, and in the process of riding my bike, I was hoping to heal my ravaged body and my wounded soul.

—ONE—
The Cradle of My Dreams

He who is in pursuit of a goal will remain empty once he has attained it. But he who has found the way, will always carry the goal with him.
—Nejc Zaplotnik

The Sava River glitters like transparent sapphire and emerald gems as it rushes from the Julian and Karavanken Alps in Slovenia. One of the longest rivers in Europe, it rises from two sources: Sava Bohinjka and Sava Dolinka. Sava Bohinjka emerges as a waterfall that cascades down Komarcha, a sheer wall below Triglav, Slovenia's tallest mountain, and the symbol on the nation's flag. Sava Dolinka lazily bubbles as a spring out of the ground in lush green meadows just a few miles south of the Italian border. Each travels several miles to join at the foot of my hometown of one stoplight and a mouthful of a name, Radovljica.

Rich in history, my town was first established in the thirteenth century, when dukes, counts, and Habsburg emperors ruled and built fortresses, castles, and churches perched on hills. Centuries of students who came before me wore down the marble steps of my primary school. On the first day of second grade, I slipped and tumbled down the entire flight, landing at the bottom. Blood streamed from an inch-wide gap on my chin, staining the new yellow dress my mother had sewn.

The natural history and the beauty of Radovljica still captivate me, but the Sava River runs through my veins. At once thunderously crashing over rocks, forcing its way through deep and narrow gorges, or dreamily meandering across soft green meadows—I am like that river. Teeming and pacific. Full of passion, pride, and quiet, heartfelt adoration for the people and places that helped me become the person who is always seeking new adventures yet craves the warmth and comforts of the familiar and safe environment.

I grew up fishing the Sava with my father's father, Toni, skipping rocks and chasing snakes with my older brother, Jure. We swam its icy waters until our bodies went numb, our lips, fingers, and toes turned blue. My life resembles this river.

Over millennia, the Sava River etched a series of terraces, slowly carving her way into the sloping hills. On the first plateau below our five-story apartment building lay train tracks. That was forbidden ground for my brother and me. The first thing we did when we came home from school was run up the four flights of stairs and throw our backbreaking school packs into the hallway. We knew our parents wouldn't be home for at least two more hours.

Often, we'd run straight to the train tracks. We could tell time by each passing train sounding its whistle while it sped by us. We'd place coins on the tracks, duck down behind the embankment, and watch the sparks fly. I'd watch people's heads whizzing by and wonder where they were going. The smell of the railroad still brings back the memory of train cars rattling by. The urge to be on that train that would take me away from home to a faraway world of imagination was irresistible.

We were fueled by book plots and our own imaginations. My

brother, a big fan of Howard Pyle's *The Merry Adventures of Robin Hood,* wanted to test his marksmanship skills on me. Imagining himself to be William Tell, a legendary hero famous for his crossbow and archery skills, Jure placed an apple on my head and ordered me to stand still against the entry door. Replacing a bow and arrow with a kitchen knife, he stood at the other end of the hallway aiming at the apple on my head. Quivering with terror, I screamed as the knife flew in my direction. The knife missed the target by about six inches and lodged into the soft tissue under my tongue. Copious amount of blood streamed from my mouth. My brother held a teacup under my chin to catch it, all the while begging me not to tell our parents.

I didn't because I couldn't talk for days afterward.

In September 1974, when I was ten years old, a famed Orient Express train traveling from Athens to Paris collided with a commuter train two hundred yards out of Ljubljana, the capital of Slovenia. It ran the red light on a foggy morning, leaving fifteen people dead and many seriously injured. The reports from state-run papers and media showing mangled steel cars and bodies didn't talk about the notoriously high accident rate of the Yugoslav rail system. I had no time to worry about such things. Agatha Christie's mystery novel *Murder on the Orient Express* sat on a nightstand next to my father's bed. I wanted to read it, but English was still unfamiliar to me.

My father read it aloud, translating for me as he went. I was captivated. I knew that if I could sneak onto the commuter train at the station near my house, I could run away to the main station in Ljubljana and hop aboard the Orient Express. I didn't tell my brother about my plan. This was going to be my own adventure. On the day my brother had a clarinet lesson after school, I slipped past the conductor and hid in the train lavatory. We were soon on our way to the grand capital of Ljubljana. But the combination of a rocking train car and the repulsive smells coming from the toilet made me sick. I got off the train at the next station and arrived home on foot just in time for dinner.

This was just the beginning of my thirst for adventure.

I next turned to my bike (which had the double the advantage of less rocking and no stinking toilets). "Franjo" was named after one of my first crushes. He was electric blue, steady, and capable of making my dreams of traveling and adventures come true. When his human namesake broke my heart, I tore the entire bike apart, nuts and bolts and other parts scattering in our driveway. I intended to paint it all a new shade of red to exorcise the pain of grade-school rejection. By then, we had moved into the house my parents built at the edge of town. When my dad pulled into the driveway after work, he just stood there in bewilderment.

"I am not buying you a new bike! If you can't put it back together, you're walking!"

I did put it back together, but several parts were still lying on the ground.

"It works!" I shouted to my father the next day when he came home from work.

Looking down at the remaining bolts and nuts scattered in the driveway, he shook his head. "It cannot possibly run!"

I proceeded to prove him wrong by riding a victory lap around our house, circling around my dad, and coming to a skidding stop next to him, my face shining.

"Will you look at that! Maybe you should be an engineer!" he exclaimed. "Like me!"

I looked away, staring at my feet, proud but shy.

During those early years of school, my dad and I spent endless hours going over my math problems. These sessions often ended with me in tears. He'd always go back to what he referred to "the basics," and we'd end up sitting there for hours. I'd stare out the living room window where a two-hundred-year-old linden tree towered over our house. I just wanted to get the damn homework done so I could go outside to climb that tree, explore the woods, or ride my bike. I knew that disappointed him. I'd always wanted to please my dad, just as later I would always want to please the men I was with, hoping to find a piece of my father in them.

When I was fourteen, my father took me to a slide presentation and lecture by a famous Italian mountaineer named Reinhold Messner. I could hardly believe that this national hero shook my hand. I still remember my tiny hand disappearing in his rough, strong grip. Messner and his partner, Peter Habeler, had just returned from climbing Everest without oxygen, something that had never been done before and was considered an impossibility. They proved to themselves and to the world that you can find a way to do the impossible. It was one of the few times in my life I was truly star-struck, speechless in the presence of this bearded giant with a thick wavy blond mane. I don't remember if he said anything to me. It was in his steely blue eyes, reflecting the mountains cased in the impenetrable ice and snow, that I saw myself. I knew then that I wanted to climb my own impossible mountain.

During my senior year in high school, my gym teacher showed us a slideshow about his bike ride through the Middle East. Inspired by him, I wanted to ride a bike across Europe and beyond. Daydreaming of riding through Turkey, Iran, Iraq, Syria, and other exotic lands occupied my mind as I stared out the window during classes. Learning about geography and history from books and listening to dry lectures could not satisfy my curiosity. I wanted to travel all around the world. On my bike. Alone! I had other lofty dreams. I wanted to be the youngest Slovenian woman to climb Everest.

Growing up in the golden era of Slovenian Alpinism, I watched our climbers returning from scaling impressive original routes in the Himalaya and being hailed as heroes. I remember distinctly the day when an expedition returned from a successful climb of Everest's West Ridge Direct. Nejc Zaplotnik, the youngest Slovenian to stand on top of Mount Everest, was a member of Kranj Alpinist club, with offices right next to my high school.

I was a member of that club as well. The Alpine clubroom was always packed with a bunch of sweaty, smelly, bearded guys—and me, a small blond high school girl. I was waiting to hear Nejc's reports, see his slideshows, and listen to his stories from faraway exotic places. After the meetings I rode home on my bike fifteen miles in the dark, often in the rain. My bible was Nejc Zaplotnik's book *Pot*, which doesn't mean the kind of pot we smoke or cook in, but "The Path" or "The Way." *Pot* still sits on the bookshelf across from my bed in the great company of books by mountain climbers, explorers, and other adventurers. In 1983, Zaplotnik died in an avalanche on Manaslu, leaving his young wife and three sons behind. In his book, he wrote a line that inspires me to this day: "He who is in pursuit of a goal will remain empty once he has attained it. But he who has found the way, will always carry the goal with him."

When I was a sophomore at the University of Ljubljana, I made a spur-of-the-moment decision to ride my bike across Slovenia. Slovenia is a tiny infant of a country, and there are a mere two million of us. We are surrounded by high mountains to the northwest bordering Italy and Austria, wine country hills spill to the Hungarian border in the east, and the Adriatic Sea splits a contentious border with Croatia to the south. The ride took only a handful of days, the time I had between classes. I did little planning, just strapped a sleeping bag on my bike and started riding. I had no trouble finding quiet country roads to ride. I met people in villages along the way who generously fed me. I drank from fountains and streams, picked apples and pears along the gravel roads, and slept in barns snuggled in hay. I tried drinking milk straight from the cows' teats, but that didn't go over too well. I was seventeen. I was full of wonder and dreams of new places and challenges. My bike satisfied my desire for freedom and planted the seed for future adventures.

A year later, at the end of the fall semester of my junior year, I boarded a plane with a backpack and a pair of skis to teach skiing for a winter in Squaw Valley, California. I said goodbye to my family. I was to be gone the whole second semester of my junior college year. I fell in love with Lake Tahoe the first day I arrived. It was Thanksgiving, the first one I was able to celebrate. I could ski powder, climb smooth granite walls, windsurf across the deep blue lake, and eat juicy turkey all on that same day.

I came to love Lake Tahoe and its surroundings. I returned to Slovenia planning to finish my studies, but as fate would have it, I would never live there again.

Toward the end of 1984, not long after I'd arrived in the States, I took a road trip with two freshly minted friends, Mike and Rob. Mike's family had invited me to stay with them in Squaw Valley until I found the place of my own. Rob was Mike's college friend. Both avid skiers and skilled mountain climbers, they were home on a Christmas break, planning to ski the Popocatépetl and Iztaccíhuatl volcanoes just southeast of Mexico City. I eagerly agreed to join them, neither considering a lack of camping or climbing equipment nor worrying about the dwindling amount of dollars in my pocket. At age twenty, one does not worry much about the future. I just knew that things would somehow work out. It was a lofty goal for a three-week trip. I was looking forward to skiing the glaciers of these two massive volcanoes and excited to explore the Great Pyramid of Cholula, the largest pyramid in the world. Our first stop was to climb for a few days in Yosemite. Looking up at massive granite walls I'd only read about and could only dream of climbing, I was in awe. It was a completely different climbing style than what I was used to in the crumbling limestone rock of the Julian Alps using pitons. Jamming my fingers, fists, elbows, and my entire body deep into cracks and chimneys was a new experience. I was a good athlete. I was light and strong and flexible, so I quickly caught on to the new climbing style. My fingers bled, but my heart sang with freedom on the rock. Mountains were where I always felt most at home and alive. I felt like I belonged.

On my first New Year's Eve in the US, we slept under Yosemite Falls as it was bathed by an almost full moon.

Two days later, I turned twenty-one. We climbed one of the all-time classics, the fifteen pitch Royal Arches on a glorious, sunny California day. The snow was melting on the ridge above us, and we bathed in water that was collecting in pools on the sheer, vertical granite wall way above Yosemite Valley. But we also lingered on top of the climb for a bit too long. We rappelled back down and landed on the cold, snow-covered ground in pitch dark, ate frozen pizza, and went to sleep.

Our next stop on that same road trip was to climb the rough granite boulders in the high desert Joshua Tree. We were having a great time climbing but realized we were running out of time to drive all the way to Mexico City to ski the volcanoes. We got as far as Mulegé, a town on the Sea of Cortez along the eastern edge of the Baja California Peninsula.

In early 1985, the Transpeninsular Highway 1, also simply referred to as Mex1, was rugged, and many sections remained unpaved. Although we were strongly advised against it, we camped on deserted beaches and drove at night, surviving on cans of beans and the youthful spirit of adventure. The boys constantly made fun of my broken English, and I was getting tired of being the butt of their jokes. One night, while camping on yet another beautiful and empty beach just south of Mulegé, we were sitting by the fire, roasting hot dogs on sticks. Listening and trying to understand the meaning of their jokes, I suddenly jumped up, feigning terror. "Someone is walking around our car!" I shrieked. Both boys jumped up, Mike holding the knife between his teeth. Both were ready to fight the invisible bandits. I smiled inwardly with satisfaction. It was payback time. Mike and Rob didn't close their eyes that night, while I slept quite soundly, curled up by the fire.

I fell in love with Baja's rugged frontier. I felt its mystical energies and the presence of ancient spirits. I knew that someday, I'd be back.

There, I felt free.

—TWO—
Changing the Course

I was born to be born, to remember the steps of all who approach,
Of what pounds at my chest like a trembling new heart.
—Pablo Neruda

Returning from Baja to Squaw Valley, I was even hungrier to travel the world and began making plans to climb and ski mountains on every continent. I also yearned to continue exploring the Baja Peninsula and the Mexican mainland.

On a very crisp morning in February, I was hitchhiking to work at the Squaw Valley Ski Resort from neighboring Alpine Meadows, where I shared a house with several young ski racers. A red Bronco pulled over, and a friendly man named Tom and his wife gave me a ride. The car quickly filled with Tom's loud and enthusiastic voice. He asked questions, and we told stories. Mostly, he told his stories. Tom worked for a well-known ski and outdoor company, and they were looking for models for a photo shoot. Always ready for an opportunity to make any kind of money that would help fulfill my dreams of traveling, I quickly accepted his offer to model ski clothing. The week-long photo shoot paid well.

After that, my path continued to cross Tom's. Not all our meetings were coincidental. Still, I had no interest in anything more than a friendship. Soon, I returned home to Slovenia to finish my studies at the University of Ljubljana. Tom was persistent, often calling me at my parents' home. He assured me he just wanted to chat, but my parents grew more and more concerned. They would warn me to stay away from a man who was much older than I and already married. During one of the calls, Tom informed me he was getting divorced. He had many suggestions about our future.

"You should come back to the States and finish your studies here," he said.

I liked that idea and started applying to different schools in California. Eventually, I transferred my credits to the University of Nevada, Reno, an hour drive from Lake Tahoe. The school offered me a ski scholarship, and Tom offered me a place to stay in his mountain cabin.

Tom started inviting me to heli-skiing trips and ski fundraising events sponsored by the company he worked for. I would meet famous musicians, movie stars, and other influential people.

This is how naive I was. In a plush ski resort in Colorado, I was introduced to Mr. and Mrs. Ford. Many of the ski events were sponsored by car companies, so I assumed Ford car company was the sponsor. I was quickly corrected that the couple standing before me were, in fact, the former president of the United States and his wife. Everyone around me, including President Gerald Ford and his gracious wife, Betty, had a good chuckle. I wanted to evaporate into the thin mountain air. Tom thought it was hilarious. I was an innocent young girl, looking for a father figure.

Growing up in a small town in what was, at that time, still Yugoslavia, I was terribly impressionable, and I allowed myself to be won over by a man fifteen years my senior. I imagined life with him would be one perpetual adventure. What I liked about Tom was that anything was possible. His enthusiasm was contagious. A born and well-trained salesman, he could talk you into anything. While his divorce was in process, our relationship grew into something more than friendship. Just before I graduated, I got pregnant. Marriage followed. We were in constant motion, soon with our first, second, and then third child in tow. My children became my entire universe. Motherhood changed me. There was no time to follow through on my plans to return and travel alone through Mexico. Climbing and skiing the tallest peaks around the world was just a wishful dream of the past. But I didn't mind. I was in love, and this love for my babies consumed me.

The nomadic lifestyle can be fun and exciting, but with three small children, it was impossible to follow a routine. I got hardly any sleep. I was exhausted. Besides our age and cultural differences, Tom and I had very different ideas on raising children, which soon became apparent. Piles of Christmas presents grew larger every year.

"We need to get away from all this stuff, Tom," I pleaded. "We need to simplify our life. I'm burned out."

The growing materialism became a constant topic of conflict, and our marriage was strained because Tom didn't seem to listen. Instead, he would show up with new cars, dirt bikes, sail boats. I needed to have a say in things but felt I wasn't being heard. This tension went on for several years. Finally, I packed a few bags, loaded the kids into the family motorhome, and drove to Baja. Our friend Bruce Spradley had told me about the Bay of La Ventana south of La Paz, a beautiful place where winds blew throughout winter. This is great place for windsurfing, which Tom and I were both very passionate about.

"All I want for Christmas this year is just to be a family," I said to Tom in as firm a voice as possible, before driving off. "We'll get each kid just one present, something they can remember."

A week later, I pulled into the campground on the beach in La Ventana. The kids ran around and played all day while I enjoyed windsurfing and the wind on my face. Like climbing mountains, sailing across the water and catching waves on my windsurf board made me feel free. There was no TV, just sand, wind, the sea, and plenty of other children for my kids to play with. Happy and exhausted, each night we snuggled in bed, and I'd read to them until we all fell asleep with smiles on our faces. I fell in love with La Ventana Bay's abundant sea life, pristine white sandy beaches, and small fishing villages on the Sea of Cortez.

Tom flew down a couple of weeks after I'd arrived to join us for Christmas. As soon as we picked him up at the airport in La Paz, and I saw the giant orange North Face expedition duffel bag bursting at the seams, I knew we were in trouble. It was full of toys I thought we'd agreed we wouldn't buy, especially electronic toys like Game Boys. In the interest of keeping the peace, I swallowed my words, but the resentment that had driven me away two weeks earlier continued to build.

We both agreed that La Ventana was a beautiful place. At the end of the trip, we purchased a piece of land two miles out of El Sargento village, where no other houses were visible around us. We planned a life off the grid that would last between Thanksgiving and the New Year. Over the following summer, I designed a simple palapa, a palm-thatched roof structure with no walls, that provided sun protection while we enjoyed the magnificent outdoors surrounding us. We were finally in agreement—or so I thought—that keeping life simple, playing board games, reading books by candlelight, and exploring the outdoors was good for us all. Baja became my safe place. I should have been happy. We had three beautiful children, a lovely home in the mountains, and a simple but beautiful place on the edge of the ocean; we drove nice cars, made good money.

It didn't last.

After I gave birth to our second baby girl, Jana, Tom and I started to drift apart. I could no longer feel the love for the man I was married to. I felt guilty and ashamed, and I blamed myself. Because the pregnancy was complicated, I'd been confined to bed rest. Terribly concerned about the wellbeing of the baby, I neglected the needs of my husband, or so I believed. Longing to free myself, I wanted to leave, but couldn't. I was too scared to be on my own with two little babies. I carried on with everyday tasks as if someone had turned on automatic pilot. There were apologies, there was remorse, there was begging for me to stay, but a large part of me died, and I was numb to any love other than the love for my babies. Not knowing what else to do, I agreed to have another child in hopes of healing our marriage. Three years later, my beautiful baby boy, Tilen, was born. My children were my salvation, and I had no room to love anyone else. There was a fundamental divide between Tom and me; a threatening, dark cloud was casting shadows on what should have been a happy life.

Still, I didn't want our marriage to end. Why else would we have bought property in Mexico? For years I held onto our marriage with everything I had. I realized more and more that I'd made a mistake or had changed. Most likely, both. I became increasingly restless. Baja was supposed to be our healing place where we could just be a family. Instead, it magnified our differences. I fantasized about leaving while the leaving was still possible.

I often thought about our pet bird, an orange-fronted conure. I named him Jaka after my uncle. I loved that bird almost as much as I loved my father's brother. After returning home from one of our many family trips, I walked into the house, expecting loud screeching greetings from Jaka. He was always so excited when we returned home.

Nothing. All was quiet.

I walked to the cage. Jaka's little, green-feathered body lay on its back, tiny feet sticking stiffly into the air. In horror, I realized I'd forgotten to ask the neighbor girl to come over to feed the bird and give it water. I was responsible for killing the bird locked in a cage, helpless, doomed. The kids started crying and ran away, but I just stared at a tiny, stiff, shriveled body and thought, *This is going to be me if I don't open the door to this cage and fly away.*

I thought of my grandfather, who suddenly lost the will to live, and how that frightened me when I was young.

My grandpa owned a grocery store, but if you asked him what he did, he'd say he was the keeper of the bees. I adored him and would sit under one of his apple trees for hours, watching bees fly in and out of their hives, each painted a different bright color. Atek is what I called my grandfather. Diabetes robbed him of his right leg when he was still in his prime. He'd often sit in a chair under the apple tree wearing his blue work apron, and we'd watch the bees together. He wore a black rubber boot on his good leg, and his crutches leaned against the back of a wooden chair. I'd rest against the trunk of the apple tree, its rough bark poking me in the back. No matter where I seemed to look, the stump of my grandfather's right leg—still purple and red from amputation—was always in my peripheral vision. It frightened me. The constantly oozing wound disgusted me, but I also found it fascinating. I could never look fully away from it. The knee was still there, a five-inch stubble dangling off the edge of the chair, always smelling of the antiseptic lotions my grandmother would apply.

"Remember this, my Lenka," he would gently lecture. "Honey, is the best medicine for everything."

Then he would spread a dab of honey over his tender red scab before continuing. "All these modern medications the doctors pre-scribe cannot compare to the magic of the nectar the bees create. Don't forget this, nature always knows best."

As he spoke, I tried to hide my tears. Every summer, as far back as I could remember, we would climb aboard his light-blue moped and ride to the forest just a few miles away from my grandparents' house in a small village called Kokrica. There, we'd pick blueberries, mushrooms, and sweet wild strawberries. My grandfather seemed ancient to me then. But he was fit and strong. He was only sixty-six when they admitted him to the hospital, after complications from his diabetes became grave.

In a postcard to my grandmother from the hospital, he wrote, "I have to make a decision which surgeon to choose. One wants to remove the leg above my knee, the other below it. I feel as if I'd been struck by lightning. I want to just come home and end it all. You should make a decision if you want to live with and take care of an invalid. Send me your opinion by whoever comes to visit on Sunday. Your loving husband, Joško."

The doctor my grandpa chose cut his leg below the knee. His leg was gone, and so was his dignity. I remember all of us piling into the family car the following Sunday. My father drove our tan-col-ored Audi. Grandma Hani sat in the passenger seat, and the rest of us squeezed into the back. My brother and I couldn't even fight. I was sitting in my mother's lap, my uncle, (my father's brother) sat in the middle, separating us, and my brother sat in my aunt's lap, (my mother's sister). Yes, that was my family. Two brothers married two sisters. No seat belts were used back then, and my parents spared us by not smoking in the car that day. Off we went to see my grandpa and the leg that no longer was. It was a somber ride to a hospital in the capital city of Ljubljana. With my face pressed against my aunt's armpit, I fought back nausea. The sweet and sour smell of fear permeated every cubic inch of the stagnant air in a car way too small for seven people.

I was a small child, but I felt even smaller in the presence of the tall gray building in which a doctor just sawed off my grandpa's leg. Walking through the white, echoing hallways of the clinic, I regretted not hiding behind the bee shed in the lush, green garden when we picked up Grandma Hani. The nurse pointed to the door at the end of a long hallway smelling of disinfectant. My brother and I made squeaking noises, dragging our sneakers in skating motion across the shiny, gray, linoleum floor. We were quickly reprimanded to behave properly, which was to be seen but not heard. We all squeezed into the room, which smelled of bananas and oranges. For some reason, they were the standard gift to bring to a patient, as if they would admit a ray of tropical sunshine into a windowless room. Every white, metal-framed bed had a gray metal cabinet next to it. Every metal cabinet held rotting bananas and oranges. There were three beds in a row on each side of the room, separated by white curtains.

All I remember grandpa saying was, "I can still feel my toes on my leg."

That was enough. I've never forgotten that ghostly image.

That day he lay in bed, listless, frustrated, sad. Starched, creaseless, white linen sheets were stretched so tight I was afraid to wrinkle them, so I didn't touch them. A light-blue cotton blanket covered both his legs, but a bump under the blanket ended abruptly on the right side. I could hear adults saying words, but they had no meaning, except that I knew they were desperately trying to cheer up my grandfather. I just stared at the void in the bed and the tubes coming from under the blue blanket, that ran to a clear receptacle hanging off the edge of the bed, into which a pungent, yellowy fluid dripped. The visiting hour was over.

"Take me home to die."

I heard the odd voice that no longer belonged to my grandpa. The room also smelled of decaying flesh and disinfectants. I now hate the smell of rotten bananas, rotten oranges, decaying flesh, and disinfectants. A few weeks later, a white ambulance with a red cross painted on the sides and blue light flashing on the roof brought grandpa home to die. All he wanted to do was sit under the apple tree and watch his bees. He didn't die. My grandma's love wouldn't allow that, even after he suffered the stroke that crippled him. He became a little child again, crying at every family meal.

The day before I boarded the plane for California, I came to kiss my grandpa goodbye. We were sitting at the kitchen table, kneading dough for pasta. Grandma, as always, stood by the stove, frying liver and onions. The smell of it watered my eyes. A red-and-yellow-colored transistor radio was playing polka music. Suddenly, grandpa burst into tears.

"I'll never see you again!" he cried. "America is so far away!"

"Oh, don't be silly, Atek! I am only going to be gone for a few months. By the time our apple tree blooms again, I'll be back!"

I was on the plane the next morning.

Only two months later, I was up in the mountains, sharing a crowded cabin with other ski racers, when the phone rang. My mother was on the other end of the line.

"Atek died this morning," she said, her voice barely audible through the tears. "I held him, and it was peaceful. Before he closed his eyes, he asked me to tell you he loves you."

I held on to the cold phone receiver, shivering. I couldn't make a sound.

The next morning, I caught a ride to the city to get off the mountain, out of the snow, and away from the pain.

I spent that night in a stranger's apartment. We made no attempt to act as though we'd ever see each other again. I quietly untangled myself from his clammy sheets and hurried into the fog-shrouded morning. My body felt wooden. Heavy. I kept moving, passing shops, noticing nothing around me. Then it hit me: the smell of roasting coffee. The very same smell of my grandpa's roasted coffee in his grocery store. It penetrated my nostrils, slid down the back of my throat, entered my lungs, and oozed into my bloodstream. In an instant, I was a hopeless heap of sobs. I crumbled onto the curb and cried until snot dribbled over my lips and down my chin. There were two halves of me now, split even further by death. One rooted in the Old Country, one looking for what was to become of me in the New World. The void would never be crossed again. People just kept walking by, stepping around me, glancing at me in discomfort. No one stopped. I was invisible in Fog City, surrounded only by air saturated with the aroma of roasting coffee beans.

I thought a lot about my grandfather in the years after my divorce. I sought solitude wherever I could find it, often jumping on my bike in search of solace. I'd push my bike over punishing hills, hoping the exertion would soothe my scattered mind and wounded heart. After one particularly grueling day, I found an apple tree heavy with unopened pink buds and delicate white petals. The branches were buzzing with bees—a hum so strong it sounded like the tree itself were trying to fly away. I found a place to sit under the branches and let the sweet air transport me back to my grandpa's garden. I thought about the abrupt change in the life my grandfather so cherished. It beat him down, leaving him unfulfilled. I wondered if my divorce would follow a similar course.

Pulling out my light-blue, pocket-sized collection of the Persian poet Rumi's work, I sat under the apple tree reading. Something in that moment inspired me. I took out my pen, turned to the back of the book, and wrote this:

"I am just trying to do things right, to live without regret. I want an adventure. The attainable kind. It will give me time to think, time to feel, time to write. Time to feel alive again. Time to be alone. I want to ride from my home in Tahoe to my palapa in Baja."

There it was, in black and white, the kernel of an idea that would forever stare at me whenever I'd opened that book of the great Sufi poet and philosopher's work. It was more than just an idea. It was an inner command, pointing me toward what I needed to do. Finally, I had a sense of how to connect the painful dots of my confusing and grief-ridden life, but life was busy, and the years kept going by, the dream tucked away for that someday.

—THREE—
Ready to Love Again

To love:
to create a body from a soul,
to create a soul from a body,
to create a you from a presence.
—Octavio Paz

No divorce is ever amicable. I don't believe the process is easy for anyone, no matter how ready they think they are. In mine, there was a lot of confusion, sadness, bruised egos, and blame. Blame for quitting the marriage ultimately fell on me. We were on Christmas break in Baja when we told the kids we needed to separate for a while to figure things out. We all sat on the bed in the family motorhome.

"Your mother has something to say to you," Tom said to the kids.

I clenched my fists and looked out the window, holding back the tears. At that moment, I hated Tom even more for placing all the blame on me in front of the kids. Even as the words came out of my mouth, I couldn't believe I was saying them.

"Your dad and I need a bit of time apart."

Tom sat on the bed looking at me with his arms crossed, stern eyes, lips pressed into a tight line. Mateja, our eldest daughter, sat up straight and said, "Do us a favor please. Don't drag this out and keep us hoping it will all work out. Just get divorced and move on. It will be easier for everyone."

She was fourteen, and she was holding the hands of her eleven-year-old sister, Jana, and her seven-year-old brother, Tilen. A floodgate of tears opened, and the three of them were swimming before me. But watching them hold hands gave me hope that they would get through this together. Mateja watched her best friend's parents go through a lengthy divorce and knew how difficult it had been for that family. The girl and her two sisters resented their parents for giving them false hope. Still, I was broken and feeling incredibly guilty, watching my beautiful children and feeling their pain. They didn't deserve this. But staying together for the sake of the kids didn't feel like the right thing to do any longer. I was thirty-nine and dying inside. I didn't believe in living falsely. We decided Tom would fly back to Tahoe with the girls, to get them home before school started. At San Jose del Cabo airport, I hugged the girls tight but couldn't hold on to them forever. Tom handed me his wedding ring without looking at me and walked away. I wanted to say I was sorry, but it was too late for that. It was too late to say anything. I had long ago reached the point of no return. My love for him died a long time ago, and I couldn't find the way back to what I thought love meant to me when we first met. I needed to rediscover who I was beyond my role as a mother and a wife. That day I stood alone at the curb of the air-port, teetering on the precipice of the unknown and uncertain future. Tilen's little blond head was looking out the window, his eyes following his sisters and his father walking away. He was too young to understand what was happening. Everything was blurry. I held Tom's ring, then removed mine from my right ring finger and slid both into the pocket of my shorts. I climbed into the thirty-eight-foot monster of a motor-home and started my drive north. Finally, I had made the hardest deci-sion of my life. Frightened but emboldened with the prospect of new beginnings, I flew the safe nest. Eventually we came to an agreement that Tom would keep the mountain home; I would keep the palapa in Mexico where I felt free, safe and happy; and, for the time being, we would share the motorhome.

A few days later, on January 5, 2002, I pulled into an RV park in Truckee. The temperature was four below zero. The kids weren't excited about living in a freezing motorhome in winter. I was looking for a house I could afford to buy with the divorce settlement. In March, we moved into a small fixer-upper cabin. I was elated to be free of the bonds of the unhappy marriage. For the first time in my life, I had a house of my own. It had no foundation and was poorly insulated, as it had been built for summer use only. It didn't matter how small and shabby it was in comparison with the house I'd left; for a long time, that house had not felt like home.

Soon, I was overwhelmed with juggling work and a busy life with three kids. I tried to immerse myself in painting and fixing up the small cabin to create a new home for the kids and me, but I was depressed. I'd drop the kids off at school in the mornings, come back to an unfamiliar place, and lie on the couch, trying to harden myself. But I couldn't. I was paralyzed, unable to do anything until I had to go back to pick the kids up from school. Our seven-month-old golden retriever, Bodie, lay on the couch next to me with his head on my lap while I tried to unclench what felt like the grip of an iron collar around my neck. Without judgment, he was patiently waiting for the fog to lift from my brain and my heart.

One night after the kids had fallen asleep, a bottle of Chardonnay empty on the coffee table, I went for a walk down to the lake. Losing my footing on a wooden bridge, I fell several feet, landing on the rocky ground below. I woke up shivering with no idea where I was or how long I'd been there. I wanted to die.

A shooting star split the night sky and jolted me back to reality. I thought of my children, alone in an unfamiliar house. They had named it "the House of the Ghosts." They referred to the room they shared as an orphanage. I ran back to find all three of them sleeping in my bed. Hungry for their warmth, I slipped under the covers and gathered them in my arms like three little kittens. I listened to their soft breathing and made a vow never to leave them alone again.

In the summer after I moved into my own house, I went on a mountain bike ride with a man named Jim whom I had known and had a crush on for years. We got lost and had to hike out carrying our bikes on our backs up a steep and rocky hill. When we got to the top, we sat down on a flat granite boulder, the sun warming our sweaty backs. Suddenly we both started laughing. We wondered how we could have been so lost. As we sat in silence looking across the lake, he turned to me and said, "I will never hurt you."

Years earlier, I'd met Jim in front of his brother's house. I was there to pick up my kids from a playdate, and he was standing next to a snowplow. The snowbanks were still over five feet high that spring. Jim held a golden retriever puppy in his arms, which were the size of two snow shovels. His daughter was holding onto the belt of his Carhartts. Jim was gentle with the puppy and his shy daughter. My kids and his brother's kids all gathered around the two of them, petting the puppy. I wanted Jim to pet me with his large hands. I wanted him to hold me as gently as he held his puppy. I wanted him to place his hand on me, to comfort and protect me. All I saw were his hands and his piercing blue eyes. It was not the first time I regretted being married. But I held on because we had kids. I believed that you must hold onto marriage no matter what when one has kids. And now this guy with his blue eyes and a puppy was standing in front of me, smiling at me shyly, not saying a word.

Years passed. The kids grew, and so did my unhappiness. Jim kept showing up in my life. Usually, I'd see him at dinner parties at his brother's. But he appeared in my dreams as well. All I could do was think of him. I'd never felt that way before, and I was sure I was going mad. I would be telling myself it was just my mind trying to escape the life I was living. But all I wanted was to spend every waking and sleeping moment with that man. The man who had a daughter. The man who was not the father of my kids.

The first time I asked Jim what he wanted in life, he gave me a very simple, one-word answer so typical of him.

"Home."

The meaning of everything I yearned for was wrapped up in that one word. I pushed him for more.

"What does that mean to you?"

I waited eagerly for his explanation. He didn't think for long.

"Love, family, flowers on the table, aroma of fresh bread baking in the oven, watching the snow accumulate so we can go skiing, fire in the stove to keep us warm, sitting next to you reading the Sunday paper, dog by our feet."

That was one of the longest string of words Jim had ever put together without taking a breath. It was enough for me. He promised he would never leave me, but it would take years to learn to trust again. How could anyone promise something and remain true to it?

When we started dating, it was like two meteors colliding, sending sparks into space. I was afraid our relationship would evaporate when the passion cooled down. I was worried we'd both end up hurt again.

Jim was an exceptional athlete. On his mountain bike, he would clear huge jumps that I was way too chicken to attempt. While back-country ski touring, I'd fall behind with a whimper on the uphills, unable to keep up. On the downhills, he struggled to keep up with me, though. I was a better skier. He loved playing hockey with his brothers and friends. He was a champion Laser class sailor. Together we loved cross-country and back-country skiing, ice skating, wind-surfing, kiteboarding, paddle boarding, sailing, hiking, and running. Actually, no, he hated running, but sometimes he would come along just to appease me and would run a few strides behind me as if he were my personal six-foot, two-inch bodyguard.

Six years after my divorce was finalized, Jim and I got married on top of a mountain, on the flat granite boulder overlooking Lake Tahoe. It was the place where we were lost and found on our first mountain bike ride together. On a sunny day in March, we climbed up the mountain on our skis. Surrounded by our family and friends, the big blue lake, and the snowcapped mountains, we each made a promise for the second time in our lives *to have and to hold from this day forward, for better, for worse, for richer, for poorer, in sickness and in health, to love and to cherish, till death us do part.*

I slowly started moving our things to Jim's house six months after we got married. I kept my house for a few years just in case. Jim had been a bachelor for fifteen years after he divorced. It was like going from zero to sixty overnight, once I moved in with three kids in tow. It took years of adjustments to turn his house into a home for all of us together. In time it became an oasis where he and I could both retreat from the world.

—FOUR—
Perfect Storm

Acceptance of the unacceptable is the greatest source of grace in this world.
—Eckhart Tolle

In January 2016, I was working as a ski team supervisor at Squaw Valley. I knew the mountain well.

Skiing has been my life ever since my father put me on a pair of sky-blue wooden skis with yellow plastic bases and screw-on edges that were perpetually rusty. ELAN was printed on the tips in red letters. Elan skis, the pride of Slovenia, are produced in the factory I could see through our kitchen window. I was fiercely proud of the connection.

When I was very young, my father would strap my black leather, lace-up boots into spring-loaded cable bindings and pull me up the hill in front of our house until I was proficient enough to sidestep it myself. Snow would stick so thick to the bottom of the yellow bases that I'd be almost as tall as my brother, who was a year older. When I'd crash going over the jumps my brother and I built, the skis would break, but never would they release from my feet. Instead, I'd crash and then stand up, covered in snow that stuck to my royal-blue, cable knit, wool sweater, cherry-red wool gloves, and matching red hat with a giant pom-pom that my grandma Mira knitted. I'd shake it off and hike back up for more on a broken ski, limping through the snow like a wounded animal. Our noses and cheeks would be red from the cold, and our hands and feet would be frozen. But we wouldn't come home until Mother called us for the third time to come inside for dinner.

I was a competitive ski racer in Slovenia. I competed through college and spent years following the best extreme skiers in the world on one of the greatest ski mountains. I'd never been seriously hurt.

Besides training coaches and overseeing the groups, my role at Squaw Valley Ski Team was to take over for any of our Big Mountain Ski team groups when needed. On a particular day, one of our coaches was complaining of neck pain, so I took over her group of kids after lunch. A blizzard raged around us, and half the mountain was already closed. I took the group to a slope where I thought the visibility and snow might be better. As we prepared to take our last run of the day, I was looking forward to handing the kids back to their parents and getting out of my cold, wet clothes. I already pictured myself sitting by the warm fire, snuggled next to Jim, holding a glass of wine in my hand.

A strong gust of wind brought me back to reality on the mountain. I was scanning the slope below me. Accounting for all eight kids in the group, I sent them down the next stretch of trees and then followed. I could hardly see through the curtain of falling snow and blasting winds, when I nearly collided with a small tree. To avoid it, I quickly turned right, but the tips of my wide powder skis were buried, so the right ski didn't follow my body. I heard my knee audibly snap.

Instantly, I knew I was in trouble.

My knee was dislocated, and as I tried to release the binding, I felt it pop back in place.

Shit.

I was flat on my back in the cold snow, unable to move. I checked my phone. No signal! I reached for the two-way radio on my chest. "This is Mothership; anyone on Shirley Lake? I need a ski patrol. I'm in the trees on the second tree run directly below the ski patrol shack." I yelled at the kids to stop, and miraculously they heard me. "You have to hike back up; tell the rest of them," I called to the nearest one. The others were barely visible through swirls of large snowflakes. "You're in charge. Keep everyone together and wait," I told the boy closest to me.

Soon, another coach arrived. "Ski patrol is on the way," he said. "I'll take the kids down."

"Eight of them, make sure you have all eight of them," I said and closed my eyes again, on the verge of passing out.

I lay in the cold wet snow, looking sadly at the pair of Elans still attached to my feet as I waited for the ski patrol. As I tried to process the pain, I realized that the young child's ligaments and bones are much more pliable than those of a fifty-something-year-old. I was still making peace with that realization when I looked up to find two handsome young ski patrol guys standing over me.

"How are you doing, ma'am?" one of them asked.

Ma'am? Did this guy just call me ma'am?

The thought that I might look that old made me groan. Hot tears of pain flowed out of the corners of my eyes and collected in the edges of my ski goggles. Some of them escaped, running into my ears. I was freezing. The pain made me want to puke.

His next question was even worse. "How old are you, ma'am?"

I wanted to punch him, but I just lay there on my back in the cold snow.

When I replied, "I'm fifty-two," I shocked even myself.

Fifty-two? It sounded like someone else was talking. It was the first time I heard myself say my age out loud since my birthday on January second, only a few weeks earlier. I was in my blue-and-white coaching uniform, bundled up with a neck gaiter, goggles, and a helmet. *Do I really look old enough for this guy to call me ma'am?* I wondered. "Just get me off the mountain, please! I don't really care about anything else right now!"

By the time I got to the medical facility, I was shivering, and I was in shock. The patella of my right knee was dislocated, and an MRI later revealed that I'd ripped most of my ligaments, torn my meniscus, and bruised my tibia plateau. Reconstructive surgery was scheduled. My ski season was over and, as it later turned out, so was my thirty-year coaching career.

A few days after reconstructive surgery, I went back for a checkup to get the metal clamps out.

"How is your pain?" the doctor asked.

"Not bad. I still can't feel my leg."

"Oh, that's not good" the doc replied after a moment of silence.

"What do you mean? Isn't it good that I don't feel much pain?"

"No," he said carefully. "What I mean is it's not good that you don't feel anything. The sensation should have come back by now."

During the anesthesia and a nerve block, which was performed without ultrasound guidance before my surgery, the anesthesiologist damaged my femoral nerve by inserting the needle too far into the nerve. My leg finally started waking up, but the damage had been done. It was waking up with a vengeance. The whole upper part of my leg was hypersensitive for several months. Nothing, not even a bed sheet could touch it. It was agonizing, my quad spasming and cramping continuously. I couldn't get any sleep. Jim couldn't get near me except to hold me in his large arms at night and comfort me.

With everything we had been through, our love ran deeper than ever, but talking about hard stuff has never been easy for us. Whenever the word *communication* is brought up with Jim, he wants to run as fast and as far away as possible. He is a master of redirecting a conversation if it doesn't suit him. All too often, when I say things to him, I'm met with silence. Jim's childhood friend Dana nicknamed him Dropped Call. He has met with silence so often when they talk on the phone that Dana thinks Jim is no longer on the other end of the line. If I say, "Please say something," he will reply, literally, "Something." And then I want to reach up and rip his heart out.

After the surgery I was laid up on the couch in the living room, hooked up to an ice machine. Clanking of dishes and plates and muttering came from the kitchen. Jim was searching for the items I'd apparently hidden from him when I moved into his house eight years before. I'd taken over the kitchen, but first I had to rid the drawers and cabinets of Jim's work tools and sawdust. He didn't complain. I love to cook. Food connects us, and sharing meals with family and friends makes us feel at home wherever we are.

After the surgery, I was in pain and immobile, so Jim was in charge of cooking. He would bring me scrambled eggs, toast, and tea on a tray just the way I liked it. Dinners were a simple affair.

On the fifth day he asked, "Feel like taking over yet?"

"Oh, you got this, Jim. You're a great cook."

"Yeah, right. You better get back in here, or we'll both starve to death. I miss your cooking."

I told him it was good to practice. One never knows what's coming. "Besides," I said, "I like it when you cook for me. Makes me feel loved."

In April, while I was still hobbling around on crutches, my parents arrived from Slovenia for my daughter Jana's college graduation. To celebrate, my parents, the girls, and I flew to Baja for a week

before the commencement. My son, Tilen, was busy with his finals.
Jim stayed home with our dog, Monty. Happy to be out of the snow,
I was watching the sunrise from my bed under the palapa. The red
cardinals, bright yellow hooded orioles, and different varieties of
warblers were jumping from gnarled branch to another on a *torote*
tree right in front of my bed. I could smell the briny ocean and the
blooming desert. Enjoying the morning coffee my mother brought
me, listening to the symphony of birds, and watching the sky change
shades of rose, I was back in my own paradise. I just happened to
reach up to my breast, and I felt it. The lump was round and hard. I
realized that this is what a breast tumor must feel like. Although I
hated myself for even thinking about it, that sixth sense, that deep
intuition made me realize that I'd been in denial way too long. I
had been noticing for a while that the shape of my right breast was
different. It looked like a zipper was pulling the bottom of my breast
up to the nipple. I justified the way my breast looked by figuring I
was getting older and should just gracefully accept it! Cancer never
crossed my mind. As soon as I felt the lump, though, I knew it wasn't
supposed to be there.

I lay in bed holding my coffee, which grew cold. The birds went
quiet. The world around me seemed to die. As the days went on, and
I sat under the sun umbrella with my leg propped up next to my parents on the beach, I'd watch my daughters playing in the ocean just
like they did when they were little girls. I tried not to think about the
lump. I kept my suspicions to myself. My daughter was graduating. It
was her celebration, her achievement. I didn't want my mother and
father worrying.

As soon as we returned home to Tahoe, I made an appointment
with the doctor who had delivered my first baby. I watched his
expression when he performed a physical exam and looked over at

the nurse. Stone-faced as he always was, he couldn't hide it. I knew it. He knew it.

"We need to schedule a mammogram and a biopsy," he said matter-of-factly. Then he grabbed his clipboard and hurried out. The nurse quickly followed. Something was terribly wrong. Neither the doctor nor the nurse made eye contact with me as they passed by the examining table where I sat in a stupor. Knowing my doctor for years, I could feel the shield of self-preservation going up around him. It was as if both of us knew what the tests would reveal. The lack of words and face devoid of any expression spoke volumes.

The doors shut behind them, and I was left cold and alone in the room with walls painted in soft pastel colors, which are supposed to be soothing. The water from the silver faucet was slowly dripping into the sink. My butt was stuck to a piece of white, glossy paper on the table. A blue paper gown was draped over my shivering body. I looked down at my breasts, which were covered in goosebumps, the left one nice and firm, the right one sadly drooping, the nipples hard. I suddenly started shivering, realizing all at once that my days could be numbered. All my unfulfilled dreams could go up in smoke. I dressed up in a hurry, grabbed my bag and my crutches, and hurried out of the office without stopping at the front desk.

The nickname "Mothership" suits me well. I kept the news to myself. I felt I needed to protect everyone around me, including— perhaps especially—Jim, until I was certain. If it turned out to be nothing, I felt it wouldn't be fair to make him worry about me. And worry he does. Obsessively, especially when he doesn't have all the facts.

I used to be a sales rep for outdoor clothing lines. On one of my business trips to show my product to a buyer for Yosemite retail operation, I ended up spending the night in the hostel just outside of the park after my long day of appointments. There was no cell phone reception for me to check in with Jim that night. I had another appointment the next morning with an account in Mariposa, a town just outside Yosemite National Park.

As soon as I arrived, the owner of the retail store said, "You need to call your husband right away. He is very worried about you." She handed me a landline, as my cell phone still didn't work.

"How did he get your number?" I asked, incredulous.

"I guess he called your company."

By the time I reached Jim at nine in the morning, he already called my kids. They had no clue where I was, since they were staying with their father. Jim had already filed a missing person report with the police and the highway patrol. That incident alone made me think I wanted to wait as long as possible before I gave him the news about the cancer.

So, instead, I told him I had to have a preventive mammogram, and they were just doing some further checking. I didn't want him to worry prematurely. And because I've always been a counselor for other people's troubles and afraid to show my weakness, I didn't ask a friend to take me. Instead, I drove to the Reno diagnostic center by myself. There, they stuck a long, thick needle into my breast to cut out a tiny chunk of the tumor, so they could send it to the lab. As I drove back home, my breast felt as if it were on fire. I was scolding myself for not asking someone to accompany and drive me.

Waiting for the results was excruciating. My gut told me it was not going to be good. I bided my time through my daughter's graduation. I said goodbye to my parents as they returned to Slovenia. I prepared for my son's twenty-first birthday.

On June 8, 2016, at exactly three in the afternoon, my cell phone rang. I was working downstairs, packing orders for Tahoe Teas, the organic tea company I'd founded soon after Jim and I were married. I had always dreamed of owning my own business. I was behind on deliveries to my accounts. Although anxiously waiting for the phone call, I hesitated for a few long moments before answering.

"I am sorry to give you the news, ma'am. The tests of the biopsy are positive. You have an invasive ductal carcinoma."

Motionless, I was staring across the yard through the glass door when a small bird suddenly thumped into it. I watched his tiny lifeless body fall out of sight. The voice on the line brought me back to reality.

"Ma'am? Are you still there?"

The doctor explained what ductal carcinoma was and told me he had already notified my surgeon, who would be calling me shortly. I would later learn that the tumor was nearly thirty millimeters, and cancer had spread to two of my underarm lymph nodes. That meant that cancer cells were floating around within the lymph system and could have already spread to other parts of my body. The doctor first recommended surgery to remove the tumor and the tissue around it. Radiation and aggressive chemotherapy would follow, as well as targeted medication therapy to block cancer cell growth.

The doctor droned on, saying that the results of my treatments were uncertain. I would become a statistic and forever hope that cancer didn't suddenly show up somewhere else. Only time and symptoms would tell. As he continued his patient explanation, I could only think of how many women this poor doctor has had to call.

"Thank you, Doctor," I said as if I were swimming underwater. I promised to think about it and call back.

"Yes, we will need to make a decision sooner than later," he said.

Still sitting at my workbench, I was breathless. Inhaling suddenly as if I were coming up for air after a deep dive in the freezing lake, I

slowly slid off the chair and retrieved the crutches. I hobbled across
the room toward the door, holding a silver door handle, feeling its
coolness. Across the yard, the soft green leaves of a vine maple tree
fluttered gently in the afternoon breeze. I held my breath and then
finally, ever so slowly, opened the door and lowered my gaze. The
body of a tiny gray chickadee with a soft white belly, its head bent
at an odd angle, lay on the black doormat. A small droplet of blood
at the edge of his beak stained his silky white collar. I kneeled and
scooped up the lifeless but still warm body. His wide-open black eyes
stared up at me, as if to ask, *What just happened*? I made a little ham-
mock with my sweater, dropped the bird into it so I could hold my
crutches and the sweater with one hand, and carried him to the vine
maple. I dug a shallow hole with my fingers. I liked feeling the pain,
digging into the hardened soil. Gently placing the tiny body into the
hole, I watched it for a few moments before covering him by scraping
the soil into a little mound. After placing a few rocks around and over
the top, I stood, tearless, watching my little bird's grave.

I limped to the front of the house. Jim was in the driveway, talking
to a friend. I was not ready to say anything, trying to delay his pain. I
was still processing my own shock about the news, but he just looked
at me with his striking blue eyes. Deeply intuitive, he knew that
something was amiss.

"Well?"

"Not good." That was the only answer I could muster for him.

We hugged, and I got in the car and drove to the post office like
I did every day, got the mail, and went to sit on the edge of the vast
blue lake. The mountains surrounding it were still covered in snow. I
closed my eyes, and only one thought went through my head: What
now? How do I tell my kids?

My son's birthday was just two days away. I was painfully aware that he would have a very different twenty-first birthday experience than I did thirty-one years ago. A profound feeling of guilt and pain surged through me. I had no control over this. Much as I wanted to, I was not able to protect my children from painful news.

Friday night, June 10, on Tilen's birthday, Jim, Jana, Tilen, and I went to our favorite restaurant for dinner. My elder daughter, Mateja, lived in Austin, Texas, so she couldn't join us. Since each of the kids turned ten, we've celebrated their birthdays at Christy Hill in Tahoe City. It has always been their rite of passage. We polished off a nice bottle of wine, and then Jana took her brother out to a few more bars to celebrate. In the morning, I made breakfast, and once I managed to get Tilen out of bed to the table, his face turned green upon seeing eggs sunny side up. He was too hungover, and the worst was yet to come.

I got Mateja on Skype, and now I had all three of my kids together. I broke the news as gently to them as I could, but I also got right to it.

"I know it's early, but there's no good time or easy way to say this. I have been diagnosed with breast cancer."

All was quiet. I told them what the surgeon and coordinating nurse at the cancer center had told me the day before. I was very matter-of-fact and as calm and strong as I could be, but the kids all started crumbling before me. It was hard for me to stay composed, but I had to. I am the one who must be strong for them. I am the one who protects them from all the harm in the world. I am their mother.

Tilen reached over and put his hand on my leg; I hadn't been aware that it was bouncing nervously. I looked over at Jana while tears quietly rolled down her cheeks. Mateja, the ever pragmatic and optimistic one, said, "Mom, the tests from the tumor biopsy will come back negative, and you won't need chemo. You'll get to keep your hair."

I had Tilen and Jana right there next to me, and I could hug them. I was able to assure them that things were going to be okay. Mateja was all alone in Austin. Her boyfriend had packed up and moved back to Reno just a week earlier for work. She had nobody there to comfort her. I wanted to transport myself there to be with her. Tilen got up from the table to head back to bed. He never touched his breakfast.

"C'mon, you're late for work!"

"I'm not going!"

"That is not an option! Life goes on for everyone, no matter what!" I told him.

Jana and her boyfriend drove off to work as well.

The dining room remained quiet for a long time.

The next two calls were to my brother and my parents. I was spent.

Recovering from my ski accident suddenly took a back seat. I was still on crutches, in loads of pain and discomfort, but that was not life-threatening. My world was spinning out of control.

Once I got sucked into the system, surgery and treatments followed very quickly. First the tumor, along with a good portion of my already small breast, were removed. Then they installed a port in my chest, which would later be used to administer chemotherapy. The bulging port stuck out two inches to the left of the sternum, an inch below my clavicle bone, right on the edge of the V neckline. It looked angry: purple and red and covered in small bumps. I nicknamed it Buddha and drew a smiley face on it with a marker, so I could talk to it. I was still working hard at my physical therapy for my leg, and I was driving back and forth to the University of California, San Francisco Medical Center for more poking and probing and testing to try to figure out the extent of the nerve damage of my leg in hopes of seeing some progress. All the doctors could do was prescribe more drugs. I was on such a high dose of muscle relaxants that my brain was shrouded in fog. I was unable to do much more than sit in a chair and stare across the room. My Tahoe Tea business, which I had been painstakingly building for eight years, came to a halt.

On August 2, I received my first round of chemo. That morning, just as I entered the Gene Upshaw Cancer Center in Truckee, I started my period. It was to be the very last period of my life. I felt as though my womanhood had abruptly ended.

Sitting in a reclining beige leather chair watching the nurse prepping bags of solutions, I was surrounded by a group of well-wishing friends, so many, in fact, that the nurse finally asked everyone to leave. Suddenly I was all alone and relieved to be so, watching clear liquid slowly dripping into my vein through my Buddha port. I surrendered to the drugs to do their job, contrary to everything I ever believed. In the past I'd fought taking Advil for a headache. Not that long before, I had told my acupuncturist that if I ever got cancer, I would treat it naturally with food and homeopathic treatments, meditation, and positive thinking.

The surgeon, whom I knew from skiing, said to me on the first day I came to her office, "You can do all that, but this is not the time to experiment. I hate to tell you, but a lot of people who decide to go with 'the natural treatment' come back a year or two later, and the cancer has spread so much that we can't do anything about it."

With every chemo round, my body grew weaker. I had terrible throat sores. I developed lymphedema in my right arm, which swelled to resemble a tree trunk. My nails blackened and separated from my fingers and toes. Food tasted like cardboard. Even water was tasteless. I got several tooth infections and needed emergency root canals. Reaction to antibiotics made my body swell like a blimp. All the drugs and chemicals they were putting into me were in contradiction to my fundamental beliefs. Tahoe Teas was based on a healthy balanced lifestyle philosophy: "Play, Laugh, Love, Share, and Drink Tahoe Teas" is our motto. All that suddenly went out the window.

I tried forcing myself every day to go on walks around the block in our subdivision. The narrow roads connect small cabins in our neighborhood. Lake Tahoe slowly changed colors and moods below me, distracting me from my pain and nausea. I daydreamed of getting on a bike and riding toward Baja, away from the doctors, treatments, and, especially, the bottles of medications that stood in a neat line like soldiers in orange uniforms with white caps, saluting me every morning when I entered the bathroom. Most walks, I'd have to sit down on a rock by the side of the road to catch my breath. Bodie, my thirteen-year-old golden retriever, stopped and lay down beside me. We looked at each other, and I felt a surge of conviction.

"Someday," I said through gritted teeth, "I am going to ride my bike to the end of the earth."

To this day, I am not sure quite where those words came from, but I know without a doubt that I meant them more than nearly anything else I have ever said.

My faithful dog listened patiently.

When I rounded the corner toward home, I ran into a friend. I could see in her eyes the fear and pain she felt for me. I smiled and hugged her, trying to put her at ease, and I graciously accepted a casserole she offered. I had no appetite for any kind of food. But food means comfort, and friends have the need to ease your pain when you are sick. Casseroles were stacking up in our refrigerator. One day I opened the door and couldn't find space for another of our neighbors' casseroles that had been left on our doorstep.

I found this sad and humorous.

"Maybe I should plan my own wake," I snapped sarcastically to Jim.

He didn't find it funny. Not one bit.

After another walk, I practically crawled back to the house, collapsing on the couch. I was defeated.

Jim came home, and I made myself get up and walk to the kitchen to make him lunch. I put on my brave smile for him, wanting to show him that I was not yet completely useless. After lunch, we both started sweeping—Jim outside on the deck, and I in the kitchen. I was leaning on the broom more than pushing it. He was sweeping furiously. It looked like we were both trying to sweep all the shit out of our lives.

I made neat little piles, and before I had a chance to clean them up, our younger dog, Monty, came bounding in, scattering them. It was the last straw, and I collapsed in a heap of tears.

How many times can I sweep up all this mess? How courageous am I now, staring at death?

Monty sat down beside me on the floor, placed his silky-soft, bear-like head in my lap, and watched me patiently with his warm brown eyes, then licked my tears. *Don't give up*, he seemed to be saying. *You'll be on your bike before you know it.*

In September, we had a family head-shaving party on our deck, drinking tequila and taking turns using a hair buzzer. A few days before, I'd started noticing my hairbrush was getting full of my long blond hair. To get ahead of the game, I wanted to buzz my hair super short. Surprisingly, I was excited about that. I always wanted to see what I'd look like with hair a quarter of an inch long, but of course I never had the guts to do it. Mateja, who had just flown home from Austin for her birthday, wasn't ready for that. She stood with her arms crossed, watching from a distance. I saw her tears welling up and could feel her pain and confusion.

I never thought I'd belong to any tribe and certainly never wanted to belong to the tribe called cancer patients. I was an oddball in high school. When other girls would talk about clothes and boys, I'd be out running, riding my bike, and getting in shape for skiing and climbing. But this cancer tribe? I was sucked into the vortex suddenly, swiftly, in one singular motion.

I had been stripped of everything down to my bare, smooth skin. I mean naked, shiny, white, glow-in-the-dark skin. I had more hair when I was born. Have you ever seen yourself completely bald? No hair on your legs or arms, no hair under your armpits, no eyebrows. No stray hair on your chin you secretly pluck in a car at the stoplight, hoping no one is watching. The craziest thing of all was that I had no pubic hair. Besides not having to shave my legs, I never had to worry about a bad hair day. My hairbrush lay abandoned in my bathroom drawer. I would stand in front of the mirror at a Buddhist monk looking back at me. When even my buzzed hair started falling out in clumps, my friend Doug offered to shave my head, and he allowed me to shave his head in exchange out of sympathy. We sat in the yard. Jim, Doug's wife, Laura, and the dogs watched as Doug ran a razor over my head, lathered with shaving cream. With every pass of the blade, smooth white skin appeared. My eyes were closed in surrender. It was as close to a religious experience as I have ever had.

It was strangely liberating not having to worry about my hair. I tried wearing a wig, but that would crack me up! It just wasn't me. To lighten my somber mood, Jim would dance around our bedroom with the blond wig on. He looked like his sister Diane's twin. When my head was cold, I'd wear hats knitted by friends. For the most part, though, I wore nothing at all. This is who I am now. Yes, I have cancer, and I accept it. This too shall pass. I comforted myself, embracing my new look. Yet often, I'd stare at myself in my mirror's bald reflection and wonder how Jim really felt about it. He didn't say anything.

He knew he might inadvertently hurt my feelings. It had happened before. A few years earlier, we were getting ready to fly back East to Massachusetts for his niece's wedding. I'd borrowed a couple of nice dresses from a friend, and my hairdresser gave me what she called a "sassy haircut," a medium, chin-length, layered bob. When I came home, Jim looked twice, which surprised me. He usually didn't even notice when I got my hair done.

"Like my haircut?" I asked, full of expectation, happy with the new look.

"It'll grow back," was his reply.

I just stood in a doorway, the bags of groceries getting heavier in my arms.

"It's fine. It's fine," he backpedaled.

"Fine is not exactly a compliment."

Not too many words were spoken at dinner that night. I retreated into my own world, wanting to ride my bike as far away from him as possible.

—FIVE—
Murphy's Law

Anything that can possibly go wrong, does.
—John Sack, journalist

As 2017 was coming to an end, I had already met my maximum out-of-pocket insurance deductible. I'd never had a colonoscopy, so I decided to schedule one since it would be covered. Just a routine checkup. Two nurses, who were also my friends, wheeled me out of the prep room.

"See you in a few minutes!" I called back to Jim, who was standing, slumped over, watching me disappear into the procedure room. More than two hours later, they wheeled me back into the recovery room. I was still groggy, and Jim was sitting next to me when the doctor came to talk to us. He sat down on a stool and rolled over to my bed. He reached for my hand. Well, that's unusual! I thought. He went on to explain that he'd removed many polyps in several sections of my colon, but many polyps remained. He referred to it as a carpeting of polyps, also known as Gardner syndrome, which is a genetic syndrome causing colon cancer. He was drawing a picture on a pad, as if I were in an anatomy lecture.

"Most likely, we will want to remove at least those sections of your colon," said the distant voice coming somewhere through the fog of my brain, "but first, we have to send the polyps to be tested for cancer and wait to make a decision for treatments."

I'd just received a second death sentence.

My already groggy mind could barely process the diagnosis. Jim and I both cried along with the nurses around us. I was already searching for the words to tell the kids that I had colon cancer as well. I was still bald as a cucumber from my first chemo rounds, which were not yet finished.

As I slowly got dressed, I thought, *I guess this is it, the end of it all.* The end of my life was all I could think about. How could I possibly survive *two* bouts with cancer?

What followed was a seemingly endless cycle of more tests, waiting for results, and more uncertainties. My life became a regimen of endless trips to UC Davis for genetic testing and to see gastrointestinal specialists. *This is excruciating,* I told myself. I soon learned I had no idea what that word really means.

The winter of 2017 brought the largest recorded snowfall in Tahoe. Fortunately, Jim had a snow removal company. It was one of the few bits of serendipity that occurred during those years. He would be out clearing snow on the roads in our subdivision day and night. It had snowed for days without a break, throughout January and February. We couldn't even see out the windows because our house was buried beyond the roof. If Jim wasn't out on the roads for hours straight, he was in the garage fixing broken equipment or towing out cars stuck in snowbanks. Although I was finally free of crutches, my limp was still very pronounced. I was still weak from chemo and radiation, but I carried on like a trouper, shoveling the decks, cars, and paths around the house all day long. As soon as I was finished clearing everything, I had to start all over again because it had snowed another two feet.

Jim is a very quiet person, but, as preoccupied as I was with myself, I saw he retreated inward even more. He was constantly complaining of stomach pain. I'd been noticing a tremor in his right hand when he would accompany me to doctors' appointments. I was convinced it was all related to his hard work and the stress we both were going through.

One morning in late February, I walked into the living room to find him staring into his computer, cold white light casting shadows on his face. Without turning in my direction, and in a barely audible voice he said, "I think I know what I have. I think I have Parkinson's."

The silence lay heavy between us.

The third time was not the charm.

I was standing in the kitchen in a pair of blue-and-green-striped wool socks. My grandmother Hani had lovingly knitted them for me years ago, and now they kept my feet warm. The vertical grain fir wood floor was scratched by years of wear and tear and the dogs running across it. Usually, I could glide in my socks from the kitchen to the living room, but now my feet felt trapped in concrete blocks constructed by Michael Corleone's thugs, who were ready to plunge me into the depths of Lake Tahoe.

The room around me shifted. My feet went numb, and I slumped onto a chair next to the dining room table. I ran my fingers across the indentations of the letters and numbers the kids had made over the years, bearing witness to endless hours of homework and many family meals we had shared. My gaze froze on a tree growing through an opening cut into the middle of our porch. A double glass sliding door separated my chair from a squirrel dragging a pinecone to the gap between the deck and the tree. The pinecone didn't fit.

As much as I wanted to deny it, I knew that Jim's simple statement had forever changed our life together. But I couldn't say that out loud.

"I'll call for an appointment right away," I said instead. "I'm sure it's just stress."

By then I was on a first name basis with every nurse, and we got an appointment for the following day. We both were still numb. During our seventeen-mile drive into Truckee, I told Jim it would take a long time for any confirmation of Parkinson's, but to my surprise, we walked out of the office with a handful of pamphlets and an appointment for a brain scan. All the symptoms we had been noticing now made sense. Jim was a competitive Nordic skier. In the last couple of seasons, his right ski pole had been dragging in the snow during his swing. He was working hard on improving his technique, but the drag of the pole was getting worse. Every night when he was drifting off to sleep, his arms, legs, and sometimes his whole body would be jerking with surges of energy. Often in the middle of the night, he would kick me or punch me when his overactive brain wasn't able to separate dreams from reality. I would have to gently wake him up, and then we both would lie there stunned. He would apologize over and over. I would just hold him, and we'd comfort each other until we were able to go back to sleep. We'd also been noticing his speech was affected by his facial and tongue muscles seizing up. He was extremely upset. Often, he would just sit in his chair and burst into tears. My big, strong, beautiful man was crumbling before me.

More testing, more waiting, and the world seemed to be disintegrating around me. At home, I felt the walls closing in. I wanted to run away, but I was now managing Jim's appointments and navigating the health system all over again.

Most of all, I wanted answers I knew we'd never get. Neither of us had ever really been at the doctor's office before all this. We were athletes; we lived active, balanced, and healthy lives in beautiful Lake

Tahoe. After years of rebuilding our lives together and creating a new home for us all, everything seemed to be slipping away. In a hurry.

Somehow, one gets up the next morning and goes on with everyday life. We tried to get our heads around his diagnosis, not comprehending the full meaning of it. I would stare at the screen on my computer with words like *resting tremors, slowness of movement, loss of balance, daytime sleepiness* swimming before me. All were devastating for an athlete like Jim whose life was centered on sports and the outdoors. But words like *hallucinations, delusions, depression,* and *dementia*? Those things were unfathomable. How long would it take before I slowly lost the love of my life? We pretended this giant pink elephant did not live in our cozy mountain cabin. One day in the middle of March, we drove to town to get mail at the post office and do some much-needed grocery shopping. It had stopped snowing that morning, but clouds still pressed heavy and dark against the surface of the lake, which was inky purple and turbulent with east winds sweeping across its surface.

Just as we returned to the warmth of the car, my phone rang. I pushed the speaker button on for both of us to hear. My doctor didn't hesitate.

"The cancer panel recommends a total proctocolectomy"

I asked what that meant.

"It means the removal of the entire colon, including the rectum since you have polyps in that part as well. Those cells, which we tested, are not cancerous yet, but it is just a matter of time. It is the only way to prevent cancer."

Jim and I heard the voice on the other side of the line, somewhere far, far away.

"So, I'll be wearing a shit bag for the rest of my life?" I asked the doctor.

"We can talk about all that when you come down next week," she answered.

I thanked her, as if she had done a favor in delivering more devastating news, and then hung up.

How much bad news can one person absorb? I wondered. *What's next?*

Rather than feel sorry for myself, which was never one of my life tactics, I felt a steely resolve rise in me.

Turning to Jim, I blurted out, "I can't do that."

He nodded and stared out of the window, trying to comprehend the news.

"I want quality of life, not quantity. Whatever life I have left, I want to live it the best I can. I don't want to chase this and spend my time in hospitals and in treatment. I've lived a great life. I have no regrets."

He leaned over, placed his large hand on my trembling leg, and burst into tears.

The force of his emotion shook me. I realized he needed me more than ever—and I thought of my kids, my parents, and my yet unborn grandchildren. I wanted to be around for them. I decided it was worth anything.

Pre-op was scheduled for June 2, my daughter Jana's birthday. The gastrointestinal surgeon decided to perform one more detailed colonoscopy on May 2 in hopes that she only had to remove sections of the colon instead of the entire organ. We spent the night before the procedure at our dear friends' house in Sacramento. Suzanne drank white wine. Jim and Tim drank beer and ate sushi. I was guzzling gallons of prep fluid and running to the bathroom every five minutes, getting ready for a colonoscopy.

The next morning, it took five nurses to finally insert a needle into my veins that were already so compromised by all the chemo. I told the fourth nurse not to worry.

"I'm used to it," I said.

Then she gave up, too. Jim, who hates needles, turned green. I told him to leave the room before he passed out.

Reluctantly he did. The procedure took more than two hours, and afterward, we went back to Tim and Suzanne's house to rest for a bit.

We decided we needed a break from all the drama. We both wanted life to feel normal for a while. Our good friend Ryan, who lives on a sailboat named *Soul Rebel* in the South Pacific, invited us to come sail with him. We both needed to recharge so we could deal with questions of life and death. After paying for all the medical procedures and numerous tests, I had enough free air miles on my credit card to fly us to an atoll called Tikehau, where Ryan had anchored his sailboat.

At five o'clock on the afternoon of my procedure, we were on a sixteen-hour flight to Papeete on the island of Tahiti. We then transferred to a smaller plane to a coral atoll, Tikehau. There was plenty of time to rest on both flights.

We landed on Tikehau in the midday heat and took a five-minute walk from the one-runway airport in Tuamotu village to a small lodge, Relais Royal Tikehau. It was to be our home for two nights before we boarded the boat. A group of six bungalows sat on the bank of the river of a private motu, a reef islet formed by broken coral and sand, surrounding an atoll. When we arrived, we were welcomed with traditional flower leis and a ukulele song performed by one of the cooks. The sweat was running from our bodies in small waterfalls and collecting into tiny puddles at our feet, still clad in heavy shoes. The river was shallow, connecting the lagoon to the open ocean. The owner of this small resort showed us to our simple hut on stilts. The deck hung over the water. "Is it safe to swim?" I asked the owner as I took in the views,

"Oh, yes," answered Monique in her thick French accent. "Just a few sharks, but they won't bother you. They don't like people. We feed them food scraps from the restaurant next door, so they hang around."

"Want to go for a swim?" I asked Jim excitedly.

He refused. The sharks were huge. There was no way in hell he was going in. I told him Monique said they weren't dangerous—that she wouldn't have told us that if she didn't mean it. But he was firm.

Alone, I walked to the dock and stood on the edge, nervously looking into the murky water, dark shadows darting below. The air was hot and the water irresistibly inviting. I took a plunge, headfirst into the ocean river. It took me a moment to adjust to the light and my swimming goggles. The dark shadows scattered. I was nervous. I took a stroke and a breath, then another, and another. My body relaxed into the rhythm, and I could feel the tension and exhaustion melting away. I swam a mile without being bothered by the sharks. As soon as they sensed my presence, they darted away.

That night we had a lovely dinner on the deck of the restaurant next to our bungalow. Tahitian music, mixed with the clanking of pots and pans and plates coming from the kitchen, was a perfect background for our romantic evening. One of the staff came to clear our plates. She threw all the leftover food right over the railing into the waters. Jim and I watched a feeding frenzy below. The water was boiling with sharks of all sizes.

"You are fucking nuts to swim in there," he said, shaking his head.

I told him he was right. It is one reason he loves me. Inside, I agreed with him. But after everything I'd been through, looking death in the eye so closely and so many times, I had become immune to fear. The closer I got to danger, the more alive I felt.

* *

On the morning of the second day, Ryan picked us up in a dinghy, and we boarded his beautiful schooner.

Tikehau has an oval-shaped lagoon with only one passage, which is deep and wide enough to sail through when the tide and currents are just right. For that reason, it is rarely visited by other sailboats. We had the entire 180 square miles of the lagoon to ourselves. The atoll consists of two islands with pristine pink sand beaches. Apart from some fishing shacks, the northeastern island is mostly uninhabited. We sunbathed and swam naked. We made love in the shallow water of a solitary cove. A juvenile shark came within a foot to inspect us, then quickly darted away, but Jim scrambled out of the water, breaking all records.

According to a study by the conservationist Jacques Cousteau, that lagoon contains a greater variety of fish species than any other place in French Polynesia.

"This is paradise." I said to Jim before diving into warm, soothing waters for yet another long swim. There, I could be alone. As always, it was in solitude where I was able to be closest to myself, to my own feelings. Once in the warm salt water, I found liberation. I swam effortlessly free of the crutches, painful treatments, and endless doctors' appointments.

The atoll is surrounded by a coral reef. The islets are separated by ocean rivers flowing into the lagoon or out of it, depending on the tides. We could swim or paddleboard on the rivers for hours watching the most incredible variety of underwater fauna. Hundreds of blacktip sharks and manta rays darted through crystal-clear waters. I was so mesmerized by it all that I'd forget to breathe when I was swimming, following all the fish. I felt like I'd returned to the ocean and become a fish myself. My strength was slowly returning. At one of our favorite moorings, I swam from the sailboat to an abandoned fishing shack in the middle of the turquoise lagoon and practiced yoga while Ryan went spear fishing, and Jim stayed on the boat reading. As I watched him from the water, it looked like a photo from a travel magazine. This ought to be a custom-made vacation for an experienced sailor and sailboat racer like Jim. But it wasn't. He was nauseated from the new Parkinson's medication and fully absorbed by the shock of his diagnosis and what lay ahead for him. He was severely depressed.

Watching him not being able to enjoy our beautiful surroundings made me sad. I tried to just let him be, but it wasn't easy. I wanted him to enjoy himself, be happy and excited. I was angry too. This was supposed to be a break from all the drama and heartbreak we'd been experiencing.

I tried to soothe him with the fact that we still had each other, we were still here.

It was little comfort.

Eventually, we realized that he was seasick on the sailboat, which was in constant motion. I had some nausea medication leftover from my cancer treatments, and they soon made a huge difference in how he felt.

Two weeks into our trip, I received test results and a report from the colonoscopy. During the procedure, the doctor was able to remove many more polyps, and his recommendation was to defer removing the colon and try to manage what polyps remained by repeating colonoscopies and deciding in a year. It was the first piece of good news in months.

"I'll have a colonoscopy every month if I have to." I said to Jim. "I want to keep my guts."

Swimming alone, far from our boat, far from the shore in the deep dark waters of the South Pacific, I was surrounded by hundreds of sharks swimming just a few feet from me. They meant nothing to me.

I was living on borrowed time, and I didn't care. Nothing could hurt me anymore. The only question was, what would I do with that borrowed time?

—SIX—
El Triumfo

The most difficult thing is the decision to act.
The rest is merely tenacity.
—Amelia Earhart

At the end of 2018, we decided to spend our first full winter in Baja. I couldn't ski or coach anymore. Jim decided to quit the snow removal business but would keep his summer excavation company. We both needed a break and time to recover. With the help of my son, Tilen, daughter Jana and my friend Marilyn, I could run much of my tea business from anywhere, as long as I had Wi-Fi.

Our friends Blake and Maggie flew to the airport in Los Cabos to ride the Cape Loop of the Baja Divide. Blake was an endurance mountain bike racer who had talked about riding the 1,700-mile Baja Divide from San Diego to La Paz. The route is on dirt roads that travel through remote ranchos and fishing villages, traversing every major mountain range in Baja California. It crosses the peninsula from the Pacific Ocean to the Sea of Cortez five times. He described the ride as very strenuous, requiring a very high level of fitness and experience. There are two- to three-day stretches where riders carry all their own water and food. One must travel very light. The temperatures varied from freezing at night to well over a hundred degrees during the day.

I listened, transfixed, and thought about the promise I had made to myself in the back of my pocket-sized book of Rumi poems. I now had that many more reasons to follow through on the idea of the bike ride from Tahoe to the tip of Baja.

One of the considerations that had always stopped me was the dangerous prospect of riding on the Baja Mex 1 freeway. I've lost side mirrors to cars passing me too close; I've seen dead bodies, burned cars, and mangled big rigs on the side of the road; and I've hit many potholes the size of Slovenia. There was a white cross, decorated by plastic flowers on nearly every turn. It is white-knuckle driving. I'd driven that road many times in our thirty-eight-foot motorhome, with kids in the back watching videos, reading, or playing cards. Every time a big rig sped by, I'd be hanging onto the steering wheel, motorhome swaying left and right, holding my breath and hoping we didn't die. One time on our drive north, I was pushing my luck. It was dark already, but I had to make it to Guerrero Negro, where we'd planned to spend the night. A huge semi was barreling toward us. I pulled to the right as much as possible, knowing there wasn't any shoulder and at least a two- or three-foot drop, and clipped a cement road marker. My mother, who happened to be sitting on the toilet at that moment, came rolling out of the bathroom on her knees with pants around her ankles, screaming, "Oh, Jesus, Mary, and Joseph help! Help! We are going to die!" Then she cursed at me in Slovene, like it had been my fault.

"*Pička Materina! Jebemti koza!*" In Slovenian folk language that means, "Mother's vagina and you fucking goat."

Somehow curse words always get lost in translation. My mother doesn't curse unless she thinks she might be dying, which turns out to be quite often. She crawled on her knees to the passenger seat and just sat there, muttering curse words over and over, staring into the darkness ahead. Eventually, I had to remind her, "You might want to pull your pants up, Mom." We finally looked at each other and started laughing uncontrollably. I had no place to pull over for several miles, and when I finally found a place to stop and walked out to inspect the damage, my legs were shaking. The whole bottom side panel of the motorhome was gone. Just a black gaping hole in its place.

At first, I had thought riding across Baja on dirt roads and through the mountains was unthinkable. I thought people who do that kind of stuff are just plain nuts. But then I remembered what I had written some fifteen years ago, and I started asking myself if I was only a person who dreams and talks about doing something or if I was a person who has the guts to follow her dreams.

Who am I truly?

For once in my life, am I going to be that fourteen-year-old girl again, the one who wanted to climb her own impossible mountain? Riding a mountain bike on dirt roads and trails instead of busy and dangerous Mex1 might be an attainable goal. The huge issue was, how would I get my husband to go along with this crazy idea? But the biggest worry I had was whether I had the stamina to endure the physical and psychological demands of a ride that long. My body had gone through so much and was severely weakened and compromised.

In March 2017, shortly after my cancer treatments ended, my friend Allie and I drove down the Baja Peninsula in her Westfalia Eurovan. During the darkest hours of my treatments, I had greatly looked forward to the trip. Jim was worried sick about us back at home. We were out of touch for only one day when we didn't have cell reception. We reached Guerrero Negro, and when we finally had cell service, my phone started dinging with messages. *Ding, ding, ding . . .* all of them from Jim. I called him immediately, and the phone barely rang when he picked up.

"For Christ's sake! Where the hell have you been?" he screamed into the phone. Allie and I looked at each other in shock. For some reason, it was hard not to laugh, but I felt Jim's pain.

He was beside himself because he thought something must have happened to us. He'd been calling everyone to ask if they'd heard from us. He was just about to call the embassy to learn if they'd heard of any accidents. He was so upset he could barely talk. One of the symptoms of his Parkinson's is that his facial muscles seize up, especially when he is stressed. Also, he worries obsessively, another manifestation of both the disease and the medications. And I completely understood. Even under normal circumstances, when your mind starts going in a direction that something is wrong, it is tough to turn bad thoughts off, especially at night. I felt terrible that I'd put him through such trauma.

"I had no idea he was so worried," I said to Allie after hanging up the phone with Jim. We were sitting at a roadside taco place in Guerrero Negro, eating fish tacos.

"I don't know, Len," said Allie, licking her fingers, after squeezing lime over her taco "It's a bit much if you ask me, you know, his reaction. I mean come on, one day, we were out of touch one day."

"I know. I don't think he has control over this behavior. If I didn't know he had Parkinson's, it would really bother me, like he needs to have control over me. You know what's weird? At home he hardly says anything, like he doesn't care, isn't interested in anything I do. Then, when I go away, he's all over me, calls me all the time." I took the last sip of Corona, which by then was lukewarm and tasted like piss. "I worry about him. What if something does happen to me? This cancer shit can kill me. How is he going to handle it?"

"Want another beer, Len?"

"Yeah, I could use another one, but one is my limit. Damn! I wish he didn't worry so much. He's a tough nut to crack."

Allie is one of those rare friends who will just listen, never judge.

"It just makes it that much more difficult because we are both such stubborn and independent people."

Preparing for this ride really made me wonder what I was doing. It felt so selfish. But I realized it could be my last chance to follow my unfulfilled dream. I'd comfort myself that, for now, Jim could still take care of himself and make it through for a couple of months on his own. The uncertainty of what was ahead was telling me, *Now is the time! If I don't go through with it, I'll resent myself—and I'll resent Jim if I give up the dream that had been in me for so long, just to protect him.*

My mind was a battleground. The yin and yang pulled in opposite directions. Jim and others suggested I at least ride with other people, but I couldn't think of anyone that I could or would want to ride with except Jim or my kids. That wasn't possible. I knew Jim wouldn't want to do it, but I had to ask him. Truth be told, I wanted to do it alone. I just simply needed to do something by myself, for myself. I needed this to be my own healing journey.

Just as I started writing down my thoughts and plans, Jim came to sit next to me in our oversized chair in the office. Now what? Do I hide what I was writing? Do I hide my plans from him? I just started looking into this.

Opening the Baja Divide website on my laptop I said nonchalantly, "Wow, this site has a lot of great information."

No response.

"Want to watch a cool video?"

No response for a long time.

"Humph, what is it about?" he finally replied in his gruff voice. He was getting annoyed with me. I was like a little red ant crawling up his leg, but I needed to hear his thoughts.

"Riding bikes down Baja Peninsula on dirt roads."

Five minutes, but I could feel his mind churning.

"Would you want to do that with me?" I finally broke another long silence.

Another five minutes until he grumbled, "What would you want to do that for?"

"Well, why not? Besides, I didn't ask you if you wanted to do it, but if you wanted to do it with me. It would be an adventure, something we could do together."

"Didn't we just buy the van so we can have adventures together?"

"Yes, but this would be different."

Then I threw in for good measure, "You're the tough one, not me," which of course was true. Too often while on a long bike ride or on a long backcountry skiing trip with Jim, I would fall behind with a whimper, not able to keep up on the climbs. I'd often cry and curse under my breath, "Never again am I going with you! I can't keep up." He was one tough dude, and his reputation preceded him.

Nonplussed, Jim went back to reading his paper. I went back to looking at the website. We didn't talk about it anymore. He seemed confident the idea was going to fade away.

Now that I had conceived the idea, it wouldn't leave me alone.

Jim brings me coffee to bed every morning. One morning, I said to him, "I am becoming obsessed with this ride idea. I can't stop thinking about it!"

"Don't worry. You'll get over it." he said and walked away.

Perhaps the most crucial part of all this was that I felt I was in a race with time. By then, I was fifty-four, and if cancer returned and I had to have my colon removed, my time would have run out. My dreams would be snatched away, and the regret of not doing this would grip my soul. I thought of Steinbeck's words: "A sad soul can kill you quicker, far quicker than a germ."

My own motto, which I have always tried to live by, is, "If you stop dreaming, you stop living."

That's another way of saying that I deeply believed my long-awaited epic bike ride was meant to happen. Cancer gave me permission to follow through on my unfulfilled dreams.

Tilen was the first person I'd shared my idea with. I needed to kick it around a bit, test it out, see how the words tasted as they rolled off my tongue: "I'm going to ride all the way to Mexico. Do you want to ride with me?"

"That sounds great, but dangerous, Mom. Sorry, I'm planning to hike the John Muir Trail in the fall."

And that was that.

My son was planning his own adventure, and that was precisely how it should be.

—SEVEN—
Imminent Departure

Head out to sea—
Even if your own mother tells you to be afraid of the water.
—Rumi

The plan was in motion. I spent hours researching how to equip my mountain bike with camping, cooking, and navigation gear. One of the challenges I faced was that my bike was not bikepacking specific. I had a mountain bike. Purchasing another bike was out of the question. I had to modify many attachments, and because of the small frame, some of the packs had to be custom-built to take advantage of every inch of available space. I searched websites, read blogs and bikepacking-specific Facebook groups, especially the Baja Divide one. I had never bikepacked in my life. I had much to learn. My son returned from the Outdoor Retailer show with several pro deal cards, enabling me to order gear at much lower prices. When the equipment started arriving, I was like a kid opening presents at Christmas. My gifts to myself were a new ultralight tent, sleeping pad, sleeping quilt, camping stove, and storage bags that could be mounted on the front and back of the bike. I laid everything out on the driveway and the front lawn so I could practice which bags went where on the bike. No matter how hard I tried, there was still too much weight on the front handlebars. Jim walked by me many times when I had things all spread out, but never commented on anything, as if the equipment and my trip didn't exist. He still didn't want to believe I was going to go through with it.

Finally, one morning he gave in and suggested, "If you are really doing this, you have to have an emergency satellite device with an evacuation plan."

So, I purchased a Garmin InReach Mini, a satellite-connected personal locator beacon with an SOS button I could press in case of emergency. I signed up for an International Rescue and Evacuation Plan. I would be able to send texts through the beacon when I wasn't in cell range, which would be often. Another benefit of that unit was that Jim and my kids could track me. My signal would show up on their smartphone maps. They could see my exact location and whether I was moving. My bank account was dangerously shrinking.

I wished Jim would ask me about my new super light tent I set up on the front lawn, but he didn't. I put much effort collecting, organizing, and testing all my new gear. I'd go on short rides behind our house, only to return with half the bags hanging limply off the bike, zip ties broken. I sat down on the steps by our garage and stared at the bike and thought perhaps Jim was right. I had no business going on this trip.

I kept figuring things out, and by the end of August, I rode a fully loaded bike over Mount Watson to The Olympic Bike Shop in Tahoe City.

We weighed the bike, which was loaded with the gear, but only two water bottles and no food. The scale showed sixty-five pounds.

"How much do you weigh?" asked Wayne, a six-feet seven-inch bike mechanic, who was an experienced bikepacker and an avid traveler.

"One ten," I told him,

"Go home, spread everything out in your driveway on the tarp and get rid of one-third of your stuff," suggested Wayne.

"I can't do that. I need all this." I argued with him.

"No, you don't. Your bike is too heavy. Trust me," he said. "You have way too much clothing. You need one T-shirt, one pair of socks, one pair of underwear. Every ounce adds up. You'll just have to stink for a while. Go as far as cutting off half of your toothbrush handle."

I rode home and went back to work. I knew Wayne was right. There would be sections on the trip where the required minimum ten liters of water would add just over twenty-two pounds to the bike.

The next day I rode back to the bike shop. Wayne and his coworker, Carl, took me through what-if scenarios. We went over how to fix certain things beyond a flat tire or broken chain, like spokes and derailleur, replacing brake pads, and how to improvise, especially since I would be riding through remote areas far, far away from any bike shop. I was equipped with emergency spare parts and bike tools. Extra zip ties and duct tape would go a long way toward at least temporarily fixing things on the go. I would have to be self-reliant if I wanted to finish.

Wayne said a few times with an air of assured confidence, "Oh, you will have no issues with this bike! I'll bet you a six-pack you won't even have a flat!"

I just smiled. "Sure, Wayne!" But really, I thought there would be plenty of flats riding in cactus land. I hoped I'd owe him a six-pack.

I've never used any navigation devices, and I've been known to get lost on trails I ride on frequently behind our house. I quickly realized that was going to be one of my greatest challenges. The Baja Divide website had very good information on conditions of trails, roads, and details of resupply options. I downloaded the maps onto my new shiny Garmin Edge 1030 GPS navigation unit. This high-tech device had many more features than I needed, but a GPS tracking system that uses Global Navigation Satellite System was the crucial part. Microwave signals are transmitted from satellites to the unit on my bike to give my exact location. Maps and tracking work the same as the iPhone. I chose to use my iPhone only as a backup in an emergency, in order to save battery life for phone calls, emails, taking photos, books and podcasts for long stretches of the roads, and whatever writing I was hoping to do. Once the maps were downloaded onto a device, my location showed on the track I was supposed to follow, so I just simply had to follow the arrow and a line on the map. Easy peasy. *Even I can do that*, I told myself with wavering confidence. It took me days to figure out which apps and programs to use and to download the maps and all the information I needed. My iPhone, my new Garmin Edge, my cute little orange InReach Mini, my GoPro, and my computer kept crashing and losing everything I'd loaded. After hours and hours of tech support, I was ready to throw everything into the garbage.

Jim came home from work to find me sitting at the dining room table, which looked like a mini electronic store, and he laughed.

"You have a weird aura. Everything you touch dies."

"Come here. Let me touch you." I replied, exasperated.

Charging electronics on long distance trips in remote areas was yet another challenge. I had an extra battery pack as well as a small solar charger mounted on the front of the bike. Surprisingly, figuring out what trails I should follow through the California mountains turned out to be a bigger task. I had three options. The first one was to piece together sections of logging roads and single-track trails. Two of Blake's friends were developing maps to chart a mountain bike route from the US, to Canada, to Mexico. They were still a work in progress. I'd be riding deep into the woods in very remote areas away from any towns for days at the time, following maps that were still missing sections or were traveling through private lands without permission. That made me extremely nervous. Wildfires were another great concern. Several large fires were already burning out of control in California. I could get myself into a deadly situation if the fire cut me off and I wasn't able to escape. The second option was the Sierra Cascade Bicycle Route, which roughly parallels The Pacific Crest National Scenic Trail through Sierra Nevada all the way to the Mexico's border. And the third option was US Highway 395, which runs along the east side of the Sierra Nevada range. That option was by far my last and least favorite option, to be used only if snow came unusually early in September, which certainly has happened before.

In mid-September, we went to a mountain lake near our home to celebrate a friend's birthday. I decided to finally do a test ride. It was twelve miles. I was happy to arrive at the lake where everyone was already on their third beer and food was on the grill. That night I slept in the tent, which I set up next to our camper van. The temperature dropped to fifty degrees, but I was warm, wrapped up in two sleeping bags. It wasn't too bad, but I had to resist temptation several times during the night not to go sleep next to Jim in the van. He would have gotten a kick out of it, and I didn't want to give him that satisfaction. My departure was two weeks away. It was becoming more real by the minute.

I was starting to doubt myself. What if I get hopelessly lost, especially once I'm in the backcountry mountains of Baja? What about my family and friends? Society often judges a person who dies or is severely injured doing what is perceived to be senseless or dangerous. I have lost many friends climbing and skiing in the mountains. I was guilty of questioning their actions, and I understood them.

She was ill prepared. She was irresponsible. She never should have gone. She had it all, and she threw it all away. That was so stupid, I told her not to go. She should have stayed home with her husband and her kids, who love her.

The words echoed in my head.

I kept hearing my father, describing me: "You are like a young stubborn goat. No one and nothing can ever stop you!" He didn't necessarily say that in an endearing way.

I didn't want to be crippled with anticipation by endlessly poring over maps and planning routes. Planning has never been my strength. I was blindly hoping that I had the skills to figure things out as I went along.

A week before departure, I pulled up Google Maps, zooming in on the Baja Divide Trail. Not a good idea! It was daunting. There was a lot of nothingness, and Baja from above looked like Mars. Suddenly the whole trip, the entire idea seemed insurmountable. I quickly shut down my computer and walked away. If I looked at the maps any longer, I was afraid I would change my mind.

Growing up in the Alps, I was introduced to hiking by my dad at a very early age. Hiking and climbing are national traditions and obsessions. I can't count how many times I told my dad I couldn't go any farther. I would collapse in a heap of tears and sobs and often tantrums. Each time, my dad would patiently (or sometimes not so patiently) coax me just a bit farther on the trail. All our efforts would pay off when we reached the alpine hut at the top. Beautiful views, hot tea, delicious lunch, and feelings of accomplishment were the rewards in the end.

To encourage me, my dad would say, "Oh, it's just around the corner. See the top of those trees? The hut is just beyond them. Let's go a bit farther on the trail, and you'll get a sugar cube with lemon and some water or a piece of chocolate."

Later, as I started to climb mountains by myself or with friends, I would remember what my dad taught me. Break the mountain down into smaller sections and give yourself a mental goal to reach. Reward yourself with a little break when you make it. Always turn around and look back down and see how far you have come. Take in the view; take a deep breath of fresh mountain air. Enjoy your surroundings. Listen to the wind and the birds. Observe nature in every small detail. It will distract you, and before you know it, you'll be at the top. I learned that the mountains are a place to learn about life.

As I was going through my cancer treatments, I often compared my journey to a challenging mountain climb. I had to put one foot in front of the other, break it down into small accomplishments day by day. I often thought that if I could climb a mountain when I was freezing cold, with the wind blowing at a hundred miles an hour, snow and rain blowing in my face, exhausted beyond belief, I could do cancer treatments. I often felt I couldn't go one step farther, but then I always made it to the top and out alive. Surely, I could make it through another chemo treatment, another day of puking and feeling exhausted to the bone.

I told myself I had to go through with this trip, that I would hate myself if I became the person who only talked about plans. *If I don't go, I'll never know what I am still capable of. I have to do this, not to prove anything, but to be able to go on living.*

And to my husband, when he questioned my sanity: "I owe this to myself and to you!"

I was hoping I'd be able to find new strength physically and mentally. But, along the way, I would look around me and enjoy the view. I would smile despite the pain. Breathe one breath at a time. After all, life is about the journey until we get to the end of it all, and the final door shuts behind us.

I was prepared to see the new me unveil. I told myself I was ready, come what may.

On Saturday morning, September 22, 2018, less than a week before the start of my trip, I was riding on our small rigid inflatable boat on Lake Tahoe, driving to the Lake Forest dock to take it out of the lake and put it away in storage. The boating season was over; winter was on its way. It was a glorious morning. Fall was in the air, and my golden retriever, Monty, smelled it too. Sitting right next to me, he kept me warm, pointing his nose to the wind as we glided through the deep blue waters. His eyes were half-closed, and occasionally, he touched my cheek with his cold, wet nose. Monty loved riding on the boat, as did I. The sun was low on the horizon, surrounding us with a silver shimmer reflecting off the ripples on the water. No boats, no waves, just me, the lake, the mountains, and my faithful dog, Monty.

That morning, while I was taking a long hot shower, a feeling of doubt hit me like a raging river. I suddenly realized how very much I was going to miss all this. I would miss waking up next to my husband in our cozy bed, tangled up in crisp linen sheets, propped up with soft down pillows. I would miss our routine of waking up in one another's arms and making gentle morning love as we have for so many years now. I'd miss the short walk to the bathroom, the hot shower that is always available, Jim bringing me coffee in bed—the safety and the comfort of it all.

I finally called my parents to tell them about my trip, although my brother strongly advised me against it.

"Just tell them once you're done with it. You know how Mom is. She won't survive worrying about you day and night," Jure pleaded with me, and I could see him scratching his closely shaven head on the other side of the phone line, on the other side of the world.

"I have to tell them! It will be a lot worse if they hear it from another source."

My mother's response was predictable.

"Haven't we worried about you enough already? Now this? Why? Why are you doing this to me?"

I was prepared for that.

"Remember you gave me a book for my thirty-third birthday? It was called *Mana, By Bicycle among Indians,* by Tomo Križnar. Tomo rode from Los Angeles all the way to Panama. You wrote an inscription in it: *For a special reading and to inspire you! From your mother and father.* You gave me Tomo's original book as well, *On Search for Love, or Around the World by Bicycle.*"

I paused and then added, "Mom, I am only going to be gone for two months. It's not like I am planning to ride the bike around the world for seven years like Tomo did."

My father quietly chimed in, "You've just been through so much. You don't have to prove anything to anyone, you know! We love you just the way you are."

I knew, though, that if anyone understood me, it was my father. He knew once I set my mind to something, I wouldn't rest until I did it. "You raised me to be resilient, Dad. You treated me the same as you treated my brother. You took me to climb the mountains. You drove me to ski race after ski race. You always taught me to be tough, to try new things, to live a life full of adventure. You taught me to never give up!"

During my ski racing years, my mother worried constantly, especially when I was competing in a downhill event. Downhill is all about speed and is considered the toughest and most dangerous of all ski racing disciplines. I loved going fast. One time when my mother came to watch me race, I had a horrific crash. I entered the turn with way too much speed, and after I slid out on an icy part of the slope, I lost one of my skis and rag dolled into the orange retaining fence, ending up hanging suspended upside down like a helpless fish caught in a net. It just so happened that my mother was watching at that very turn. When I returned home, she took an ax and threatened to walk into the garage to destroy my skis.

"I never want you to race downhill again!" she exclaimed in near tears.

I pleaded with her. The national championships were the following week. I had an actual chance to qualify for the Olympic team. But she was insistent: she'd never watch me race again. I told her that was fine—she'd always made me nervous anyway.

I ended up winning the national title in downhill and got third in giant slalom the following week. My mom stayed home. She was able to see the results on the evening news. She was happy. I was happy. But then, as it turned out, Yugoslavia decided not to field a 1984 Olympic women's downhill team. The national head coaches didn't have faith in a small girl like me in a discipline where most women were twice my size. Fed up and disappointed, I quit ski racing the next year and dedicated my life to climbing and mountaineering. I preferred the solitude anyway.

I could relate to my mother's fears. I often worry about my kids doing something like this as well. But my mother and I were always two very different people, which resulted in many complicated conflicts. My mother should have known by then that I usually ran in the opposite direction of her advice. I could best teach my own kids by example. Good or bad, they'll figure things out for themselves.

I was going to take my ride, come hell or high water.

—EIGHT—
Should I Stay or Should I Go?

Wouldn't we rather have a destiny to submit to, then,
something that claims us, anything, instead of such flimsy
choices, arbitrary days?
—Alice Munro

The day arrived. It was a frosty fall morning on Friday, September 28, and I was up before the blue light of dawn entered our home. A waning three-quarter moon, along with Sirius, the brightest star in our sky, were rising in the east. My gear was neatly laid out on a blue tarp in the driveway, illuminated by the first light. Jim left for work early. He still ran an excavation business and was working on a lakefront property just down the street from our home. He couldn't deal with his emotions, so he just didn't. He kissed me goodbye like he did every morning when he left for work, not mentioning my departure at all. My plan was to ride my road bike with my two best friends around Lake Tahoe and over Luther Pass, a few miles south of the lake. There we would part ways, and I would continue to ride to Bridgeport, where we have an annual Burning Lamb gathering on our friends' property. There we roast an entire lamb and we feast. My son was to leave in the afternoon and follow me with the van in case I didn't make it all the way to Bridgeport, 144 miles away. I was hoping Jim would come to Bridgeport as well. The Argentinian-style asado BBQ party has been a tradition for years, and Glen picked the date that year, to coincide with my departure. I was also hoping to ride together with Jim up Tioga Pass to Yosemite, so he would at least be a part of my departure. There, I would switch to my loaded mountain bike. Jim, Monty, and I could have one last night camping in our van in Yosemite. I wanted to spend every last moment I had with them both.

"Will I see you in Bridgeport tonight?" I asked Jim as he was getting into his car.

"I'll have to see how much I can get done at work today."

"Well, okay then." I said, looking at my bike leaning against the garage door. Something was telling me he would come, but this was his way of showing he was not happy I was really leaving. I stuffed down my own feelings to keep the peace. But I was not going to give in. I've done it too many times in both of my marriages. Giving in to man's needs; always putting them first. I had to have faith that he'd get over it. *If he really loves me, he will understand how much this means to me*, I thought. Loving someone is allowing them to grow and letting them be themselves. I needed to have faith that our love was strong enough to survive. I took my chances.

I got back to packing my gear and took a final inventory. I checked off my gear list, which seemed endless. By concentrating on it, I could be distracted and not think about the quickly approaching departure and the weather. Rain and snow were in the forecast for Sunday. I had only two options: I could bail or get the hell out of there as fast as I could, before the snow shut down the mountain passes through the Sierra for the winter.

My friends Allie and Emily were on their way. For seven years, Allie, Emily, and I had run the youth mountain bike team we called

North Tahoe Bike Force. I was looking forward to starting my ride with these two awesome friends, wishing they could ride with me the whole way, but that was a considerable time commitment. Allie's baby girl, Dottie, was just three months old, and Emily's puppy, Honey, needed her as well.

In typical Allie fashion, they were late. By ten thirty, we were finally ready to hit the road. We took photos in front of our house before the departure. I gave Monty my last hug. "I'll see you down in Baja, Monty! Take good care of Daddy! I hope to see you both later, though."

At the end of the street, I turned around and looked at my home one last time before we set out on our adventure. Monty was sitting in the driveway, his head tilted in my direction.

As optimistic as I usually am, I doubted I could make it all the way to Bridgeport, in the Eastern Sierra along US Highway 395. One hundred and forty-four miles is a long way, and there were some steep, long climbs in between. I told Tilen he should be on standby to pick me up.

We swung by the bike shop in Tahoe City to fix Emily's brakes. We hadn't really started, and already we were having bike trouble. By the time we left the Olympic Bike Shop, it was pleasantly warm. Riding around Lake Tahoe is always spectacular. We didn't have to remind ourselves how lucky we were to live there. At the top of Inspiration Point, which overlooks Emerald Bay, my friend Pete surprised us by waiting for us. He waved and honked when we passed him. It gave me a burst of energy I desperately needed. I felt the love from so many people who were wishing me a safe journey. I knew some wished they could come along, but everyone had commitments. I was fortunate to be able to carve time out of my life to make this journey.

We began our first long climb. Allie and Emily, both world-class athletes, quickly pulled ahead. It was frustrating, and I was riddled with doubt about my ability to complete the trip. I was pushing my eighteen-pound carbon road bike with no camping gear and wondered how the hell I was going to switch to riding my gear-laden, sixty-five-pound mountain bike for miles up and down the hills on dirt roads and single tracks. Here I was on my first day, and my legs were burning, and my right quad pulsed with unbearable pain. But that was how I did things. I always dove into the unknown, hoping I'd somehow make things work. Come what may! I hummed the lyrics from one of my favorite love songs from the movie *Moulin Rouge!* with the same title.

As I sang the words, climbing the steep mountain road and crossing Big Meadow Creek, I thought of Jim. Allie and Emily were way ahead of me and out of earshot, so I bellowed out a promise to my husband with what breath I had left: *I will love you for the rest of my life! Just let me do this one thing for myself, by myself!*

On our ride around the lake and over Luther Pass, hundreds of obnoxiously loud motorcycles passed in both directions. It just so happens we were riding during the Street Vibrations Fall Rally weekend. Thousands of motorcycle enthusiasts gather every year in Reno for music, poker runs, stunt bike shows, bikini team competitions, lots of beer drinking, and tattooing. We were passed closely by low riders, choppers, and probably every model of Harley Davidson ever made in America. The riders were fully attired in black leather and American bandannas. Some waved; most didn't. Our insides were vibrating with every passing and oncoming rumbling motorcycle. It was a whole different world of people.

At Luther Pass, we rode the long, fast, and fun descent, then stopped for lunch at Mad Dog Café at Woodfords. Woodfords is a

California Historical Landmark, as it had been a remount station of the Old Pony Express Route beginning April 4, 1860, when Warren Upson scaled the mountains in a blinding snowstorm. I realized I was embarking on a history tour of California as well.

Jon, baby Dottie, and Emily's adorable puppy, Honey, were waiting for us. Fifty miles would have been a satisfying distance to stop for after a day of riding, but I wasn't even halfway to where I'd planned to ride. I held Dottie in my arms while I ate my turkey sandwich. She was restless, as was I. Allie and Emily loaded their bikes on the car to drive home. I was tempted to do the same. Luckily, there was no room for my bike. We said our goodbyes, and I took off without looking back.

You wanted this, I reminded myself. *Now go do it!*

I rode another forty miles toward Gardnerville, where I turned right onto US 395, a major Highway starting at the Canadian border, hugging the eastern side of the Sierra Nevada Range, and joining Interstate 15 after crossing the Mojave Desert. That was my third option, to ride to the Mexican border if snow shut down the Sierra Nevada routes. The shoulder was wide, the riding monotonous, and the chip seal surface sent vibrations through my body. No fun at all. My butt hurt. My back ached. My shoulders burned.

After several miles on the highway with big semis and cars blasting by me, I was relieved to finally turn onto the much quieter Highway 208 toward Wellington. It was getting dark, and I was nearly exhausted. Suddenly I saw a van pulled to the side of the road just ahead of me. It was Tilen. Somehow, I had not seen him pass me when I was rattling along on 395. I was still a few miles short of one hundred miles, so I told him to drive farther. We met up again at exactly the hundred-mile mark. It was dark by then. He loaded my bike into the van next to my mountain bike. My yellow-and-black carbon road bike looked so slim, elegant and light next to the obsidian-black, thick-framed, fat tire mountain bike, which had bags and water bottles hanging on every possible space. Tilen handed me a cold Coke. I hardly ever drink sodas, but at that moment, it tasted delicious.

We headed toward Bridgeport to Hot Springs Ranch. The seventy-five-acre ranch is a part of the Eastern Sierra Land Trust and is preserved and protected and steeped in the legacy of the Old West. It's surrounded by majestic peaks of the Eastern Sierra, and as the name implies, several hot springs are scattered around the ranch.

In the morning before the party started, I went back to where Tilen had picked me up and rode the forty-four miles I'd missed. I battled strong winds the entire ride, but I was determined.

By the time I returned to the ranch, four lambs, tied to the iron cross, were roasting in the traditional Argentinian asado style by the fire. Sausages, delicious side dishes, wine, beer, music, laughter, friends. My kids had all arrived. So had Jim. Jim! He'd come after all. I knew he would.

It was a feast, a celebration, and a goodbye. I reminded myself that the next day would be a big one. No wine for me. Jim finally relaxed a bit. We stood around a large bonfire, listening to a friend play a flamenco guitar. Jim was nursing his beer when I overheard a friend say to him, "You must be so proud of your wife for having the courage to be doing this."

"I am proud of her, but I'm also very worried," he replied quietly.

I left the party early and walked up to our van. It felt like I had so much to do, but the fact was I was nervous as hell about my departure.

I tossed and turned on a comfortable bed in the back of our camper van, thinking how nuts it was to trade the comfort of a camper van for a bike and a tent. Jim was right. We had just bought this van to have adventures together.

The next morning, at exactly eight o'clock, I rode off in the direction of Yosemite to cheers and goodbyes. My daughter's friend kept me company on Highway 395 for twenty-five miles as it gently climbed over a pass, and soon we were at the viewpoint looking over Mono Lake, the jewel of the Eastern Sierra. An ancient, majestic body of alkaline water that's over a million years old, with tufa towers lining its shores, Mono Lake is a resting and a feeding place for millions of birds on the Pacific Flyway. A fun descent led us down to Mono Lake and Lee Vining, where we met up with Jim, Jana, and my friend Kari, who also spends time in Baja. Kari is a total badass, the most decorated US woman in hang gliding and paragliding. She came riding toward us as we approached Lee Vining with her signature grin. Together with Jim, we reluctantly started climbing the twenty-five miles to Tioga Pass, directly into strong and gusty winds that literally pushed us backward.

So far, all this was not going well. I hadn't even started riding on my mountain bike by myself yet, and every day, I'd been pushed to the edge of my physical abilities.

Jana met us at the gate to Yosemite National Park with the van, and there we parted. I hate goodbyes, but here we were again. I could hear everyone cheering me on as I rode deeper into the Yosemite high country toward Tenaya Lake. This was it. I was riding off alone. The ride was beautiful among high granite walls, and the downhill stretches felt rewarding. Jim caught up with me in the van just as I reached Tenaya Lake, shimmering in the evening crimson light. We drove to find a camp spot, which was not easy in Yosemite without a reservation, even late in the season. We found a place just before dark, and while Jim was searching for firewood, I prepared our last supper together for some time. We ate by the fire and washed our food down with beer and a couple of shots of tequila. Monty lay between us, whimpering and chasing something in his dreams. Jim and I just stared into the flames of the fire, each wrapped in our own thoughts. I knew Jim was still hoping I'd change my mind, forget about the whole thing, and go home with him. His arms were wrapped so tight around me the whole night that I could hardly breathe.

In the morning, which was Monday, Jim pulled his iPhone out of his pocket while we were drinking coffee. "Are you sure you want to do this?" There was a storm warning. Rain and snow were on the way. He looked at me pleadingly, showing me the satellite map of the approaching storm. He suggested I postpone the ride.

"If I go home now, my ride is over." I said to him, tying my shoes.

"I can bring you back here next week."

I went back to the van and buried my face into Monty's soft fur and just sat there breathing into it for a long, long time.

Jim didn't want to help me take the bike off the bike rack, and he just watched me struggle with the weight and awkwardness of it. As I was completing my preparations, I ran an extra zip tie to secure the water bottle holder, and by mistake, I managed to run it through the brake disk, so my wheel wouldn't turn. Jim was still not saying anything, but I felt as if I could hear his thoughts: *Please don't go!*

We hugged one last time, and I rode off with tears in my eyes, not wanting to look back at him. I knew he was crying. This would be the longest time we'd spend apart since we started dating fifteen years earlier.

I pulled onto the road right into the path of a car coming around the corner from behind. The brakes squealed; the car barely missed me. It was far from the graceful departure I'd been planning. Jim later told me that my close call nearly gave him a heart attack.

I pedaled into the morning, my thoughts occasionally returning to that first climbing trip to the park so many years ago, when I turned twenty-one.

Yosemite Valley is beautiful, but I couldn't wait to get out and away from all the traffic. Lines of cars passed me, sometimes way too close for comfort. Suddenly, I found myself riding through a pitch-dark tunnel. It was like riding into a black hole, blindfolded without an end in sight. I was scared, but I had to keep moving. I had not turned on my lights, so I was invisible to drivers in front and behind me. I finally saw the end of the tunnel and survived riding through it. I pulled over at a vista point. The spectacle of Half Dome framed the valley in the distance and reminded me of one of Ansel Adams's famous black-and-white photographs, only in real time, in color right in front of me. I mounted a headlamp to my helmet and turned on a blinking red light on the back of my bike. While I was doing that, an older guy approached me.

"Man, I always wanted to do this. Biking and camping and going places, but my wife wouldn't let me. It's too late now!"

"It's never too late for anything!" I told him optimistically like some old pro bikepacker. I'd been on my loaded bike for exactly forty-five minutes.

"Where did you start riding?" he asked.

I told him I started in Tahoe.

He was incredulous and asked if I planned to ride the whole way back. I shook my head. "No, no," I said proudly, "I'm actually riding to Mexico."

I could tell he thought this was crazy. He called to his wife who was taking photos of the valley below.

The commotion began to draw a small crowd.

"It's dangerous in Mexico!" said another man standing next to me admiring my bike.

"Crazy people down there! You're not going alone, are you, honey?" said the first man. His wife stood next to him slack-jawed, in a white jacket, adorned with sparkling red, white and blue glitter that read, "I Love California."

She finally piped up, "You do have a gun, don't you, honey?"

I just smiled and saddled the nameless bike and bid them adieu. Once again, I almost crashed trying to steady the heavy weight under my 110-pound body as I rode away in a not-so-straight line. Watch out, pro bikepacker coming through!

Once underway, I wrestled with the first big dilemma of the trip. Which maps do I follow? The weather forecast was for rain and snow at higher elevations. I was already having trouble with my Garmin navigation device, which kept beeping at me, driving me crazy. I decided to follow the Sierra Divide maps, at least until I figured things out and got used to the bike and everything on it. I wasn't ready to enter the wilderness trails, following the tracks Blake's friends sent me. There would be no food resupply for a week. There would be no one else but the bears. Besides, fires were burning close by.

After fifty miles, and a hellish 3,661-foot climb out of Yosemite Valley, I crawled into Fish Camp at the south end of the park. During my climb, I rode by smoldering fires, smoke still drifting in a light breeze, making it harder to breathe. I was happy with the choice to ride on the road and not through the woods. It was getting dark and starting to drizzle. I stumbled into White Wolf Lodge. I decided to get a room and as soon as I entered, lightning broke up the sky, followed by ear-splitting thunder. Jim was right: the first massive storm of the season was rolling through. I collapsed on the bed.

Somewhere in the middle of the dark night, I had to force myself to get out of bed. I heated water in a microwave to mix a dehydrated packet of camping food for dinner and stared at all my gear scattered on the queen-size bed. I reorganized the bike, but no matter how I repacked it, I had way too much stuff.

In the morning, I woke to pouring rain and more thunder. I took time to regroup and repack everything again. Still waiting out the storm, I took advantage of having Internet access to deal with taxes and business emails. I already had a few challenging days of riding behind me, and I realized I needed to pace myself. I needed to make sure I got proper rest and replenished the calories I burned while riding. I needed to listen to my body, and I reminded myself that I was not twenty years old, not thirty, not even forty. I decided that I shouldn't push myself like I used to. My immune system was still compromised. If it broke down, I would be screwed, and my trip would end before it had really begun. At the same time, I felt the power of being alone and in charge of my own decisions.

Hell, I thought, *I can stay as long as I want! This is my time! I am in charge!*

I felt so liberated just to be able to make my own decisions without having to discuss it with anyone else. I had been craving this independence for so long.

The rain finally tapered off at lunchtime. I was back on my bike by one o'clock. It was a late start, but I managed another forty miles on beautiful quiet country roads. The bike and I glided down smooth, long hills. I paid for them by climbing out of the valleys to gain 2,536 feet.

I had come to my first real realization on this trip. I was on my own now. I could ride whenever I wanted to, at my own speed, as far as I could each day. I loved it. My butt and my legs, not so much. My knee hurt like hell, and my right quad was cramping severely as the damaged nerve was inflamed. I tried to ignore it as much as I could while my mind and my heart opened to the freedom of the hills around me. I inhaled sweet air infused with pine, manzanita, and the musty smell of the earth after the rain. The view from the top was breathtaking, and the downhills were exhilarating. My bike was performing beautifully. It felt as solid as it was nimble. We were slowly getting used to each other. It was my friend and my trusty companion for the long road ahead. I would take good care of it and keep the chain oiled, so it stayed faithful to me.

I made it to the town of New Auberry in the dark and stumbled into a tavern. I was all sweaty, and my hair was sticking out in all directions, so I was quite a sight among the locals sitting at the bar. A cold beer and a mushroom burger never tasted better. Listening to country music and watching people gather for the only entertainment in town, which is to play pool and drink beer, was oddly calming. For a moment, it felt like I was a part of their community. I set up the tent on the lawn behind the fire station. The next day, I would be off to the next unknown territory. The freedom of the road called me. Exhausted, I drifted off to a deep sleep. I dreamed I was falling. Just as I was about to hit the ground, I woke up with a jerk. I found myself sleeping on the hard ground, wedged between the sleeping pad and the wall of the tent.

—NINE—
Charging the Impossible

Go confidently in the direction of your dreams!
Live the life you've imagined.
—Henry David Thoreau

My body was stiff and my butt sore as I reluctantly saddled the bike, leaving the safety of New Auberry behind, and rode into the chill of the morning. I got a lot of high fives, waves, thumbs-ups, friendly honking horns, and smiles as I rode southward on country roads. Few cars were on the road. The people who passed seemed mystified, shooting inquisitive looks that seemed to say, "Look at that nutcase on a loaded bike."

I passed golden hills studded with oak and pine. This was ranch country. Some were neat, with wood stacked and ready for winter. Other front yards were filled with rusting cars without wheels, old farm equipment, trash piles, and pit bulls tied to zip lines barking ferociously.

Religion and American flags prevailed. Billboards and church signs reminded me that Jesus loved me. Christian music played on radios. I passed flag-painted mailboxes and flags flying over trailer homes that were bigger than the houses.

On one of my many climbs, a car drove behind me, slowly keeping pace and not passing. It was a lonely, narrow country road, and I was uneasy. I pulled to the right as far as I could, waving the car to pass, but not looking back. After much inner debate, I pulled over and stopped. The car pulled up beside me with a middle-aged woman driving. Her teenage daughter leaned out the window.

"We just wanted to make sure you were safe riding up this hill. People drive crazy out here!"

I almost cried with relief and appreciation.

Astonishingly, I began to enjoy climbing the hills. I could just put my head down and surrender to my thoughts, though the tiny flies that invaded my nostrils, eyes, and ears were seriously annoying. But moving felt good. I was cleaning out my body's cobwebs.

The bike still needed a name, but I was waiting for the right one to come to me. Golden hills on all sides, moss, and lichen-covered granite boulders whizzed by. The wind on my face felt soothing, and my sweat-soaked wool shirt dried quickly. Pure joy hit me like a bolt of lightning. I welcomed it. It had been ages since I'd felt this way. I smiled from ear to ear. I screamed and yodeled, even though the road stretched up and up again out of the gorge ahead of me. My kids used to be horrified when I'd yodel in front of their friends. They would shriek in embarrassment. I loved it.

A lightning bolt split the darkening sky, alerting me that rain was coming. I took a short break under a giant oak, leaned against its rough trunk and looked over the pastures where cows and sheep grazed. Wild turkeys moved deliberately yet slowly just a few feet from me, looking for food. Watching them, I wondered where I would be, come Thanksgiving.

I contemplated staying and camping as heavy raindrops made the first landings on the dry, cracked pavement. Dark and ominous skies surrounded me. The oak was a perfect place to linger, but I knew I had to keep moving. I packed up the rest of my lunch and pushed the bike through tall yellow grasses to get back onto the road. As I did, I also turned around to get one last look at the giant oak, its branches stretched wide, reaching for the sky. A barbed-wire fence separated the pasture from the road and had been there for so long that the massive oak trunk had grown around the wire and absorbed it into its flesh. It adapted and conquered and continued to live strong. The sight reminded me that if we stay in one place too long, we become imprisoned by it, paralyzed. I put on my rain jacket and kept riding, leaving the safety of the solitary and courageous oak, with its rugged trunk and roots anchored deep in the fertile California soil. The tree was strong and beautiful pressed against the golden hills in the background. I closed my eyes, and the scene stayed with me as I rode away.

I passed lots of roadkill. Squirrels, lizards, small birds, an owl with big beautiful brown wings that had a span of at least a foot and a half, many frogs, skunks, a raccoon, a possum, a baby deer with the mama deer a few feet away, their bodies decomposing and causing a blinding and nauseating stench. I rode by a rattlesnake, thinking it was dead. I stopped to get a closer look, and it started moving, curling its body into an angry ready-to-strike position, its rattle loud and ominous. I quickly lost the desire to camp in the fields of dry high grass. I was definitely in rattlesnake country. In one of Jim's attempts to deter me from the trip, he had given me a magazine article about a man who almost died after being bitten by a rattlesnake in Yosemite. The ploy didn't derail my trip, but it did make me afraid of becoming a snakebite victim. The fact was, I was alone out there, and if I passed out after a snake attack, no one would know or be there to help. I went over the scenarios of what happens after the snake sends venom into your bloodstream: passing out, vomiting, diarrhea, and internal hemorrhaging. Most of the time I didn't even have cell phone reception where I rode, but I did have my SOS button.

I started another climb. It went on and on and on, and suddenly I wasn't enjoying it so much anymore. I wanted to stop for the day, but I was still nowhere near any town. It had been raining off and on during the day, and my clothes were wet. I kept looking at my Garmin and maps on my iPhone; there was nothing ahead.

So, I asked my phone, "Siri, where is the nearest motel?"

She responded, "The nearest is Sierra Valley Lodge, five miles from here."

She added, "You are quite a ways away!"

Was I having a conversation with a computer, or was I delirious?

"Shut the fuck up, Siri!" I replied.

I was tired, wet and cold. I didn't need to hear that.

"Now, now," she said.

Siri didn't like it when I used bad language with her.

It took almost an hour to get to the Sierra Valley Inn, as it was mostly uphill. *Funky* was the word for this place. It was right out of the sixties, and not much had changed or been remodeled over the years. It did have character and charm. I got a discount because the sink didn't work. Gina, the owner, cooked, cleaned, poured beer, and swept the floor. The entertainment during my dinner on the porch was top-notch. Two guys sat at a nearby table, one large and bald, the other short, skinny and missing a few teeth. An old yellow lab sat by their feet under the table. They played guitars and sang classics, drinking beer and bourbon. Even I could tell they were making up some words.

They wanted to talk politics, and I tried hard not to react or get pulled into the discussion. I just quietly listened, enjoying my dinner. The tall bald man told me he lost everything in 2008, had a heart attack, and his wife had left him, taking all his money. He now collected unemployment and social security disability. His tale sounded like a country song. I resisted the urge to point out he had been criticizing the social systems now helping to support him. The short one then asked me if he could help himself to my garlic bread, as he clearly saw I was not going to finish my dinner.

His tall bald buddy scolded him, "You can't just eat someone else's food!"

"No, no, don't worry. I'd rather see someone eat food than throw it away," I said. And it was true. I left my dinner on my plate and said, in hopes I wouldn't embarrass him, "Here's dinner for your dog."

I hoped the cool old lab got his share, at least the bone. The wind suddenly picked up. I headed to my room, passing a cat sitting on the table. She looked exactly like a cat we gave up for adoption not long ago. Molly Rascal was a longhaired gray tabby. The cat followed me with its yellow eyes and a stern gaze, as if it were pissed off at me, judging me. "But Jim has terrible asthma," I tried to explain to the tabby. She wasn't buying it.

I'd had enough of the day. Fifty-five miles, over 4,000 vertical feet of climbing, eight hours in the saddle. I wanted to wash it off. There was no showerhead, just a pipe sticking out of the wall, but the flow was decent and hot. I applied olive oil on the saddle sores and took another inventory of my gear.

Gina was very kind to give me a box so I could send some things home. I gave her twenty dollars to cover shipping. I decided to send back an extra sleeping bag, sweatshirt, hat, T-shirt, turtleneck, and an insulated pair of long riding tights. My legs were thanking me, but I hoped I wouldn't regret it. I now had room for food and my backpack. My back was free, and I hoped it would relieve my back pain.

As soon as I lay down, the rain started. At first, I didn't even know what the sound was. It was like a sudden explosion, like a train was coming through my room. The motel had a metal roof. The sky just opened. When I opened the door, sheets of rain created a wind I could feel all over my body, and I shivered. Bolts of lightning illuminated everything, and thunder caused the thin walls to vibrate. I was so glad not to be in my tent: I would have been washed away for sure. I shut the door and crawled into bed. It was way too big and felt empty without Jim to cuddle with.

In the morning, after Gina served a great breakfast of eggs, hash browns, and bacon, I took off toward Sequoia and Kings Canyon National Parks. A slight mist was evaporating. The road quickly climbed, rising for the next 5,600 feet. I listened to *Calypso* by David Sedaris on audiobook, which lightened my mood and kept my mind distracted. Laughter helped me up the hill, and after several hours, I reached the entrance of Sequoia & Kings Canyon. The ranger at the gate informed me the nearest campground was three miles away and had no vacancy.

"You can try though," he added weakly. I began riding in the direction of Kings Canyon, but as I reached a fork in the road, my route took me away from the campground. I'd been so preoccupied following the line on my Garmin, I'd forgotten to look around. I tried to check the maps, and there were no campgrounds in the direction I was going for at least twenty miles, on the other side of the summit. I kept climbing, and the fog got so thick I had to turn on a headlamp, even though there was still an hour or more daylight left. It was now becoming crucial to find a place to camp.

At Quail Flat, I scrambled up the hill and found a semi-flat spot behind a big boulder and started setting up my tent. I hoped no ranger would be able to spot me. By the time I finished, it was dark, and the temperature was dropping rapidly. I was at around 7,000 feet elevation and freezing in my damp clothes. I immediately regretted sending my extra sleeping bag and clothes home. I forced myself to eat some salt and vinegar chips, a can of tuna, and sent a preset message on my mini-Garmin InReach satellite unit to Jim: Camping for the night. Everything okay.

The night was long and cold, and I heard every pop and crackle in the woods around me. My bear whistle was hanging on my bike outside the tent. I was too cold and exhausted to leave the warmth of my quilt and tent to retrieve it. I was expecting a bear to come into my tent at any moment. Branches snapped in the darkness. Before I zipped up my tent for the night, I threw the can of tuna as far away from the tent as I could and prayed. I promised I would pick it up in the morning if I were still alive. I didn't sleep much and was relieved when the sky gradually turned from black into lighter and lighter shades of gray. The forest around me started to wake up.

I managed to light my stove to heat water for coffee and oatmeal while still lying in my tent. I realized to my horror that the Starbucks packets I had brought along were decaf. I was so tired that even that didn't matter. During the long night, I kept having a dream that my dog, Monty, had left the tent, and I couldn't find him. I felt exhausted from searching for him in my dreams all night. Everything was soaking from the thick fog, and the tent had a layer of frost on it. When the sun came out, I carried all my things to a spot where I could spread everything to dry.

The ride started with a climb through majestic forests. There was a foot of snow at 7,500 feet. I was lucky the road was still open. Farther down the road was General Sherman, the largest known living tree on Earth, over 275 feet tall and around thirty-six feet in diameter. All these natural wonders were practically in my backyard, and I didn't even know it! I felt insignificant and humbled in its presence. I wondered how much time had passed since this tree was just a seedling. I touched the bark on the massive trunk. I was in the presence of the largest living tree in the world right then, right there! I could feel my spirit and my body growing stronger, being surrounded by these noble giants as I rode under their canopy. I felt loved and protected. I felt rewarded for all the hard riding I'd done in the last few days.

On the ride downhill toward Three Rivers, I had to squeeze my brakes for so long that my hands cramped. I descended the steep serpentine road winding down sheer cliffs, granite walls rising on all sides, the valley opening before me. These were not the foothills I was expecting I'd be riding through on my way "down" toward Mexico's border! These were impressively big mountains, exactly what I dreamed about climbing since I was a little girl in Slovenia and reading about our legendary mountaineers.

—TEN—
The Spice Man

I am not upset that you lied to me,
I am upset that from now on I can't believe you.
— Friedrich Nietzsche

Approaching the town of Three Rivers, I grappled with the dilemma where to stay for the night. I was looking for a wild camp spot by the river, but my body yearned for a hot shower after long, cold, and strenuous riding. It was getting late and dark, and I was already on the other side of town and running out of options. I was also very hungry. I hadn't had much of anything to eat all day, except some nuts and a couple of bars. I passed a Mexican restaurant that looked and smelled delicious. Right next to the restaurant was a small resort with cute cabins. I knocked on the door with the office sign. All was quiet and it sure looked like no one was around. Damn. I knocked with a bit more authority and then much louder. I finally heard some feet shuffling toward the door.

"I'm coming, I'm coming!" a sweet voice called out.

Juliette invited me into her home, which smelled of onions and beef stew. I told her I was alone on a long bike ride and desperate for a bed and a hot shower.

"Oh, dear," she said. "You need to be careful. My nephew was nearly killed by a car while riding a bike. He's still in the hospital."

She shuffled her feet slowly across the yard as I pushed my heavy bike.

"Dear God, honey. You look like a homeless person. What are you running away from?"

The cabin was all dolled up with lace curtains and heart-shaped pillows with ruffles. The best thing was that it had a bathtub.

Showing me around, Juliette said, "Now you know, the water has lots of minerals, so sometimes it is a bit murky, and it smells a bit of sulfur. But don't worry, it's good for you."

Music to my ears.

I took a shower, a much longer one than I usually take at home. I felt just a tad guilty, but my muscles needed it badly. Every square inch of my skin tingled and hurt, not unlike while I was going through chemo. I wondered, *Was I pushing my body too hard? Was I compromising it and stressing it so the cancer cells could move in and continue to destroy it?* I will be in remote areas, far away from any medical help in Mexico. I let the hot water run down my back and held my face up to the stream coming down like a warm, soothing, cleansing rain that made me feel reborn. I was trying to wash away my doubts. Every time I reached to turn off the faucet, I allowed myself just ten more seconds. Counting down slowly from ten to zero, I promised I'd turn the water off at zero. I stood in a mist, smelling of rotten eggs.

I walked next door to the Mexican restaurant, my legs soft as wet noodles. Able to get on Wi-Fi, I was studying my maps for the next day. When my food arrived, the couple sitting not far from me started arguing. As I picked at my food, I tried to ignore them, but it was impossible not to catch angry words, and I quickly understood theirs. The man was cheating on his wife, and she was confronting him. Soon tears followed. It hit too close to home and the emotion behind their words took me back to the end of my first marriage. I asked the waitress to pack up my remaining food to go. By the time I returned to my cabin, I had lost my appetite, so I took a hot bath instead. I was in bed by eight thirty and asleep by nine. I hadn't been this tired in a long time, perhaps ever, but how quickly we forget that. We have an amazing capacity to forget physical pain or exhaustion, but we have a much greater difficulty forgetting emotional suffering. It is sometimes impossible to get rid of.

I still have deep insecurity rooted in my painful experiences with quitting my marriage. I've tried to bury the pain into the deepest corners of my being. I think it's gone, but it resurfaces—usually in the middle of the night when shadows are dark and frightening. I spent the night tossing and turning. As tired as I was, I should have been dead to the world, but sleep came and went in short bursts. My dream world became jumbled with my half-waking state, and both were infused with sad and negative thoughts that I just couldn't shake off. When I woke up in the morning, my pillow was wet with tears. I must have cried in my sleep.

It took years before I finally got the courage to move out of the house and leave my broken marriage. Everywhere I turned, the pain followed and with it, insecurity. There were words of apologies, but the truth doesn't make it easier to understand. The truth doesn't make it easier to forgive. The only blame I accepted was for claiming my life back. I wanted to become a better person, not the one I was turning into. I needed to be that better self for the sake of my kids. It would take years to allow myself to open my heart to love again, and I still struggle with trust.

I took another long, hot shower, practiced some much-needed yoga for a bit, wrote, caught up on emails, went next door for breakfast, and then took one more glorious hot bath to soak my sore muscles. I had to check out at ten o'clock. I milked my time in Juliette's place until the last possible minute, even though I knew I should have been on the road a lot earlier.

The ride started with the road leading me around Lake Kaweah. In Lemon Cove, I pulled over as I saw an out-of-place scene: two guys from Louisiana cooking soul food on the side of the road. They introduced themselves as Spice Man and Brian. Brian was the younger one and was clearly his helper, perhaps his son, but I failed to ask more questions about who they were. The food smelled so good, and sampling it made me want to eat more, but I'd just had breakfast. Spice Man was persistent, and worked his charms with a thick Louisiana accent.

He said, "Oh, honey, you have to take some with you!"

I pointed to my bike. Clearly, there wasn't room for anything else.

He promised I wouldn't regret it.

He also gave me a gift: a bag of his special spices. He instructed me to use them on the first fish I caught in Baja.

"It will taste delicious," he insisted.

I repacked a few things on my bike and rode off, happily weighed down by Spice Man's wares: Louisiana BBQ, chopped kale salad, and fried fish. At least I knew now what I would have for dinner. I had a rule—I had to carry enough food for at least a day or two in case of an emergency or delay.

I took a left turn off the main road. The asphalt stretched ahead of me as if a child had drawn it right through the golden hills. It went up and down, left and right, just enough to not be too perfect and straight. There was nothing else in sight but hill after hill of dry grass and brush. A sign—"Springville 39 miles"—taunted me. It was eighty-four degrees, and I had two and a half bottles of water. It wouldn't be enough. I passed a farmhouse just as a car pulled into the driveway and figured I had nothing to lose.

"Hi, there! You live here?"

"Yes, we do," said a woman, taking a baby out of the car seat.

"Could I bother you for some water, please?"

"Of course," she said and turned to a girl who looked to be her daughter. "Bring her two bottles."

"How big is Springfield?" I asked.

"Springfield? Oh, it's small, around five hundred people live there."

After a pause she said, "So, you're riding all the way to Springfield? It's a long way," she said incredulously. "Good luck!"

Her daughter brought me two ice-cold bottles of water, and I rode off. As I climbed gaining more than 3,000 feet in eighty-four-degree heat, I thanked the mother and her daughter profusely in my mind.

Over the next few hours, only a couple of cars passed me. The road was quiet. Big granite boulders stood on either side like discarded toys left by a giant. Cows black as night grazed lazily between the rocks. They lifted their heads with grass hanging out of their mouths and stared at me with a blank expression as if they were also wondering what the heck I was doing. Wild turkeys milled about, and quail darted across the road, their feather plumes drooping in a way that makes it seem like they are always in a hurry. The sounds they made reminded me of lying in my bed outdoors in Baja, where I can hear them calling every morning: *chacuaca, chacuaca, chacuaca.* . . . .

I was becoming more in tune with my body, recognizing when I was getting tired. I stopped under a big oak to have an energy bar and some water. I reminded myself to rest and pace myself.

I had one earpiece in, as I listened to Tom Hanks's book, *Uncommon Type.* I loved his soothing yet commanding voice and his stories. As I meandered on the lonely country road, I wondered what would happen if Tom Hanks and his wife drove by in their convertible and stopped to chat.

"Where are you riding?" Tom would ask

"Mexico," I'd answer, like it was no big deal.

"Seriously?" Rita would say in amazement. "Why?"

"Oh, you know, life, cancer, and stuff! Got to do something to keep on moving!"

"You don't say!" says Rita, looking at Tom in amazement. "I went through breast cancer in 2015."

"I know! Sorry you had to go through that. It sure isn't fun! You look great, by the way!" I'd say.

"Well, you do too, honey! Keep riding! Good luck!"

Then I would ask Tom if he wants to hear what I am listening to.

"Sure," he would say. And when he'd hear his own voice on my iPhone, his eyes would widen.

"Holy shit!"

(Well, I don't know if he'd actually say that. Tom Hanks is a classy guy.)

Full disclosure: I don't follow the celebrities' lifestyles, but I just happened to have read about Rita Wilson's cancer while sitting in my chemo treatment chair. Sitting in a hospital while fighting death gives you full permission to read *People* magazine.

Anyhow, I rode with this fantasy for a while. It kept me occupied, and it kept me going up yet another hill without end. The mind wanders into funny places when you are riding a bike by yourself. You may even meet Tom Hanks and his wife Rita.

I had been on a remote road all day, feeling a bit lonely. I started talking aloud: I wished Jim were with me! He would have had fun. Well, maybe not fun, but he'd love riding on the quiet, narrow country roads, discovering new places. I missed him so much that tears started to gather in the corners of my eyes, and that made climbing even more difficult! The landscape was just so beautiful, and I wanted to share it with him. I felt selfish having all this splendor to myself.

After an hour and a half, I was finally over the crest, and from there, it was all downhill to Springfield. I surrendered to gravity, which pulled me toward what I hoped would be at least a campground with a shower. All I saw was fenced-off ranch land and high dry grasses. I was sure plenty of rattlesnakes were hiding in them. I coasted into town, and the inn stood so invitingly. My conscious mind told me, *You can't stay in another motel! You must camp! You are spending too much money!* But my body screamed, *You need a bed and a shower! You've earned it!*

My credit card was getting worried, but I booked a room anyway. Sitting on a soft, white bed, I ate Spice Man's food with my plastic fork, the sweet and spicy aroma clinging to my nostrils and tickling every taste bud of my parched mouth. I washed it down with a cold Corona I purchased at the bar while I was checking in. After so many hours riding through the heat, cold, soggy fried fish and slightly wilted kale tasted delicious. The Spice Man's food was as good as advertised. I took a shower, contemplated another beer, and instead sunk into bed. The pillows were soft, the sheets crisp, cool and sparkling white.

As I drifted to sleep, I reminded myself to look for a comb the next morning. I had been combing my hair with a fork for over a week.

—ELEVEN—
Losing Track

Oft hope is born when all is forlorn.
—J.R.R. Tolkien

The next morning, I realized I had lost track of what day it was. My phone told me it was Sunday, October 7. I'd been on my bike for eleven days. I couldn't make myself leave the comfort of the motel room. It had been the best night's sleep of the whole trip. *You are supposed to be finding joy*, I told myself. *This is not a race.* It was the permission I needed to sink back into the luxury of the oversized, soft, clean bed.

After a leisurely breakfast, I left Springfield at the crack of eleven. On my ride out of town, I stopped in two different stores to look for a comb. I had no luck, but I did find a pre-wrapped burrito at a gas station convenience store.

I started steadily climbing a kickass road that rose at 9 percent grade, not seeing the end. Big mountains loomed above me. Even though it was a Sunday, highway workers were removing dirt from the road. The road was flanked by steep canyon walls with dramatic rock features, and the nearby Tule River that runs between smooth granite boulders was swollen after the rains. There must have been a massive mudslide from the rain that had come roaring through here two days earlier. I kept climbing, certain I'd be rewarded again at the end for my efforts. Tiny flies buzzed annoyingly in my face, and I forced my mouth shut as I'd already swallowed a couple. I found it was impossible to climb a steep hill without being able to breathe with my mouth open.

Luckily, I had a bit of a tailwind that helped push me up the road. I reached Jim on the phone as I rode out of town. His Parkinson's was getting more acute and more painful each day. We had both been in denial of this terrible disease.

For the first time, Jim talked more openly about it. He's always been more comfortable talking on the phone. Space allows him safety. He complained about not sleeping well. He was able to say out loud that he was worried about our future. I could hear regret in his voice when he said he understood why I needed to go on this trip.

"You were right," he managed to say. "I should have gone with you."

"Plenty of time to do things together," I panted. It was hard to speak while climbing the steep hill. "We can ride every day when we get to Baja."

"I miss you," he murmured into the phone. "I love you."

I could barely hear him.

It takes a lot for Jim to say that. I missed his laughter, his spark, his corny jokes, and his dry New England sarcasm, which can sometimes burn a hole in my heart. Once, as I was still drying tears after one of his withering comments, I texted him the scary origins of the word *sarcasm,* "to bite the lip or to tear off a strip of flesh in rage." I was trying to tell him that's how I felt.

At the next vista point, I was still thinking about Jim when I stopped for a bottle of water and a banana. Like a clear painting of vivid greens, deep blues, cool grays, and glistening silvers, the widening valley, bathing in bright midday sun, lay below me. The river, paralleling a winding mountain road, was bursting down the granite bedrock, plunging down from great heights, creating numerous waterfalls, but I was too busy worrying to appreciate it. I worried about our health and our relationship. I worried about what the future held. The long distance between us increased my loneliness and my yearning for his company. Whatever it was, I wanted to spend it with my husband, whom I loved more than anything. Whatever time we had together, I wanted it to be lived well.

Deeply immersed in my thoughts, I stepped on my sunglasses while getting up to leave. I unrolled some duct tape I wrapped around the back of the frame of my bike for the purpose of repairs. I put the glasses back on. Scratched and skewed, they would have to do.

I kept talking to Jim in my mind as I rode on. *You are going to be okay; we are going to be okay. We are not going to let this disease take over our lives.* And then I cried again— and damn it!—that didn't help when I was climbing such a long, steep hill.

I kept looking for a lower gear that I didn't have. I pulled over again, leaned my head on the handlebars, and rubbed my back and my leg, which spasmed. I moaned with agony.

I started again and yelled, "Hey wind, give me a push, will ya? I will be forever grateful!"

But when I turned the corner, a strong gust hit me in the face. "Fuuuuuck!" I screamed into the wind, until I heard the echo of my desperation bouncing off the steep granite walls rising steeply along the left side of the road, and then, another wind gust swallowed it. I was pissed. But I refused to surrender. When I left home, I weighed 110 pounds. I could feel myself becoming stronger and leaner. I leaned into the wind.

"Not dead yet!" I shouted in my best Monty Python voice at the wind pushing me backward every time I rounded a corner until I finally reached Camp Nelson and was greeted by the sign:

Population: 180
Ft. Above Sea level: 4,682
Established: 1886
Total: 6,748

Camp Nelson is in the shadows of 14,505-foot Mount Whitney, the highest peak in the lower forty-eight states. The town has only one bar.

I set up the tent in a deserted campground and then rode my bike to the bar to have a beer and get on Wi-Fi. I sent emails to my parents and my kids and a text to Jim telling him where I was and that everything was dandy. The bar was filled with locals, mostly retirees. An older woman with long yellow hair, missing a couple of teeth, sat down at the counter next to me, holding onto a bottle of Bud Light with both hands, red chipped polish trying to cover her chewed up nails.

"You know, I was once abducted by aliens not far from here."

"Really? What happened?" I was waiting for the punch line of a joke.

"Don't remember much."

A long pause followed. I waited.

"I think they drugged me, but I got away, and here I am."

"You are kidding, right?" I said naively.

"Hell no," she insisted. "I was abducted, honest to goodness truth! On my mother's grave." She crossed herself. "It can happen to you. Better watch out, honey. They're out there."

Right then and there I contemplated ending my trip.

The bar was a perfect backdrop for a novel, and each character sitting at the counter could earn a place in it. I almost ordered another beer just so I could hear more stories, but I could hardly keep my eyes open. I finished my beer and headed back to my tent.

Other than the hoot of an owl and the soothing sound of a nearby creek, all was quiet. The stars shone brightly, and I watched them for a while sitting by the fire. I was cozy in my down jacket, hat, long underwear under my sweatpants, and I was tucked into my forty-five-degree sleeping quilt. I knew it would get cold.

Sleep came quickly, but I awakened early. The tent was still bathed in darkness, but peeking out of the door, unzipping it slightly, I saw soft gray light pushing the edges of the cold night upward. My Garmin said it was thirty-two degrees. Lingering tucked under my quilt, I kept rubbing my legs to create heat, trying to warm up. I'd opted for a quilt instead of a full sleeping bag in order to shave weight, but a lot of warmth escaped when I moved around at night, creating gaps. I thought I'd be riding in warmer temperatures. I needed to go out to take a leak but didn't want to leave my sanctuary. My shoulders were tight, and I realized I've been tightening my stomach muscles as well, trying to keep my core warm. Trying to relax by breathing softly through my nose had little effect. Every time I moved my right leg, it went into a spasm. My muscles, especially along the inner thigh, following the femoral nerve, cramped again, and pain pulsated through it, going straight up my spine and into my brain. The pain was so excruciating I screamed as if I was mauled by a grizzly bear. I just lay on my back panting, waiting for the muscle to relax and the pain to go away.

Calming down, I went over my options to bail on this "adventure." I was disheartened, alone, and longing for the comfort of my home—not out of weakness but out of recognition of how my near-death experiences had forced me to get my priorities straight.

I reached for my iPhone but couldn't get a signal, so I was using my Garmin, trying to zoom in and out on my maps. I wished I'd brought a paper map along! The maps on my riding computer were loading frustratingly slowly, and the screen was difficult to see without my reading glasses that I'd left in the bag on my bike. If I made it over this next summit, over to Ponderosa and then down to Kernville and Lake Isabella, I could ride to Bakersfield and take the bus back home.

I had hoped that by riding my bike, the muscles of my damaged leg would improve. Instead, the pain and cramping were getting worse. That alone was enough reason to quit. The sun finally started peeking through the trees, and the frost on the tent began to melt. The frozen grass crunched beneath my feet as I walked over to the bathroom. I had trouble starting my pain-in-the-ass stove to heat up water for coffee and oatmeal. It kept burning with high yellow flames instead of just short, powerful blue ones. After many tries, I got it working, and I even managed to start a fire with very damp pine needles, sticks, and logs. My inner Girl Scout was back in action.

I dried out the tent as best I could, repacked the bike, greased the chain, and tightened everything up a bit. A well-packed bike is like a well-rigged sailboat. One must maintain everything and take care of all the details every day. If you keep the sails well-trimmed, the boat will sail effortlessly. My bike, which I was starting to call The Beast, rode tight and was well balanced, even with all the weight on it. Going through the process of packing restored my confidence a bit. The sunny, bright morning put me in a better mood. I decided to see how I would feel when I got to Lake Isabella sixty-eight miles away.

Up we went for another 2,500 feet in time for breakfast. The air was crisp and getting colder as I rode toward another summit. Majestic sequoia, waterfalls, and sun-kissed quaking aspens passed by. The climb was more gradual than the previous day. It felt good. I was on M-90, also known as the Western Divide Highway.

As I climbed and climbed, submerged in my thoughts, I passed a red balloon hung up in a tree. It said HAPPY 50 ANNIVERSARY in big golden letters. I wondered how far the balloon had traveled. I wondered whose golden anniversary it was. I pictured a white-haired couple holding hands at a dinner party surrounded by all their children, grandchildren, and great-grandchildren, and they were happy. It's what I knew I wanted for Jim and me. I had mixed emotions. Knowing how uncertain our future was, I tried to picture us sitting at a family dinner table, white hair, holding hands, surrounded by our kids and their kids and a golden retriever at our feet.

After three and a half hours, I reached Ponderosa and kept pedaling. I pulled a U-turn when I saw a lodge with a sign that read GREAT FOOD! I ordered a Reuben sandwich big enough for breakfast, lunch, and dinner.

The lodge had Wi-Fi, so I texted with my kids. All three were telling me how proud they were for what I was doing. That gave me new energy and motivation. I didn't want to disappoint them. I feel so proud of them, of what they've done, of who they have become. I wanted them to be proud of their mom. I wanted to show them that we have to face everything, the good and the bad, that comes our way. My epic bike trip was my way to say to them: *Face adversity head-on, accept it, and keep moving forward. Life and time don't go backward. There are moments when pain is so deep, though, that you don't think you can ever survive. Never mind. Move forward again.*

Love for my kids is my most significant achievement, and no one can ever take that away from them or me. I had all three of them with me all the time. Their spirit kept me going through the toughest parts of the ride.

Back on the road, the sound of dry pine needles and oak leaves under my tires brought back more family memories. I thought about growing up in Slovenia and our numerous hikes through the woods, hunting for mushrooms with my dad and picking chestnuts. My brother and I would run and dive into huge piles of fallen leaves and swim in them. We would come home, often late because we'd been lost in the woods, to a meal my mother prepared while we were gone, smelling like the forest itself: damp, musty, and sweet. Riding on the Trail of a 100 Giants reminded me of that musty forest smell. It closed that gap between my loneliness and my family at home. And because I was finally descending, my mood was improving. I flew downhill, and The Beast and I broke our previous speed record when we hit 34.8 miles per hour. I screamed and yodeled and laughed at myself as we flew effortlessly downhill. Joy. It was such a welcome feeling. My mother would turn seventy-nine in a couple of days. I hoped I would be in range to call her.

Twilight was coming on strong. The darkness was a little menacing, which made me nervous about where to spend the night and how to get there safely. I needed to get to a lower elevation. I didn't have it in me to spend another night shivering. Even during the day, the temperature didn't get above fifty. I was hoping I'd make it to Kernville, but it was still twenty miles away, and the light was fading rapidly. I slammed on the brakes when I saw a sign for the Durwood Creekside Inn. It had been built in the 1930s to host employees of the Johnsdale Logging Company working up the hill. The original building was from the late 1800s and had been a blacksmith shop. The bravery of the pioneers had never been more apparent to me. They traveled this same route without phones, maps, food, or lodging. I was in awe.

When I pulled in, it looked like everything was closed. Then I heard a noise in a tent that had an old antique truck pulled halfway in, being worked on.

Out walked a gray-bearded man with a long ponytail and a cigarette in the corner of his mouth.

"Hello there! Do you have any rooms available for tonight?" I asked.

"Sure we do," said Eddy, the caretaker, never taking the cigarette out of his mouth.

The place quickly grew on me. It was like the ghosts of the past were calling me to stay, so they could whisper their stories while I was dreaming. The Kern River flowed below the decks, bright red apples hung from the trees, old tools decorated the walls. Eddy was restoring a 1939 Ford truck. The restored engine, which he proudly showed me, sat in the middle of his bedroom, which was crammed with his guitars and many items from a bygone era. It was cluttered, but I could tell that each piece held a special meaning for him. The truck was very rare, and as Eddy explained, only twenty-nine of that kind were ever made. Dave, another caretaker, had a 1938 Ford pickup. This place had character, and as was becoming a pattern, I was already making plans to return with Jim someday. Jim loves old trucks.

Safely tucked in a comfortable, warm bed, I thought about the next day. I would be riding toward Lake Isabella and switching to the second part of the California map on my Garmin and my iPhone. It would be a fresh start, halfway to the Mexican border. Falling asleep, I hoped that my confidence would still be there when I awoke.

As difficult as each day's riding had been, I began to fall into the rhythm, feeling a stronger connection between my body, my mind and the road. What lay ahead was still daunting, but I was doing something. I was covering endless miles and, in the process, I was discovering that—in the words of Monty Python—I was "not dead yet!"

—TWELVE—
I Am an Immigrant

If you are in trouble, or hurt or need—go to poor people.
They are the only ones that'll help—the only ones.
—John Steinbeck

Wednesday, October 10 is my mother's birthday. As soon as I left the lodge, The Beast and I began descending. I was soon riding in my T-shirt along the Kern River and reveling in the warmth of the lower elevation and the beautiful landscape. I loved it! My spirits were sky-high despite the headwinds picking up. I had to pedal hard where I should have just been coasting downhill. Why can't a girl get a break? But I comforted myself with the fact that I was finally out of the mountains. In my mind, it was all downhill to the border.

Lake Isabella was only a few miles away, so I decided to have an easy day and hoped I'd find a nice campground where I planned to regroup, recharge, and fix my damn stove. Reaching a county campground, I found it eerily deserted; camping season was long over. I kept riding around, and none of the camp spots called to me. I finally settled for one that had a giant boulder I could hide behind. I needed protection from the strong wind.

Resting by the fire for a few precious minutes, I sipped on miso soup, but soon the wind forced me to retreat into my tent. Somehow, being surrounded by the light fabric of the tent, with my belongings hanging from the rope I strung across, made me feel less alone. I had created this cocoon, which was now my home, and I was proud of it. Every item was within my reach. Every item had its use and its rightful place. It was cluttered in this small space, but it was a functional clutter. One side of my tent pocket held my Garmin Edge, and my helmet hung right above me with a headlamp attached. When the light was on, the tent glowed like a tiny crystal palace. My extra headlamp was in the other side pocket so I could quickly grab it in an emergency. I kept pepper spray and a whistle in there as well when I remembered to bring them in from the bike. Many nights I'd forget, and then I would lie awake all night cursing myself but was too tired, too cold, and too lazy to get back up to get them. For some reason, I found it less nerve-racking to be camping alone in the woods than in a deserted campground. I was more afraid of people than animals.

The morning crept in slowly, and as I waited for the sun to warm up the chilly morning air, I finally got out of the tent and tried to make a fire. It was still very windy, and the single log I had just didn't want to ignite. After I finally got the stupid stove working and heated water for coffee and oatmeal, I managed to lean on a loose board on the picnic table. Down went the stove and the pot of boiling water over my leg. It burned so much I pulled my pants off. It was a good thing the campground was empty while I ran around in my underwear. I ended up drinking coffee that really was just tasteless, tepid brown water smelling like miso soup. But the sun pleasantly warmed my muscles and bones. I sat on my Thermarest camping chair, bundled up in my quilt, letting the sun caress my face.

I was alone in a deserted campground, but the morning symphony of birds kept me company. I hoped that I'd finally reached warmer grounds. I could endure anything from there on, as long as I was not cold at night.

I dialed my mother for her birthday, and she answered on the first ring. "I just knew it was you!" my mother exclaimed. I was transported right into my family's living room. I could pretend I was eating cake and vanilla crescent cookies that she'd baked using family recipes passed down to her by her mother. We'd drink wine and Turkish coffee. It made me happy for a minute but also even more alone. I missed my family terribly. I was only twenty when I left home. At the time, I wanted out of there so badly. I had no idea the price I would pay. Now I was forever suspended between two worlds, never completely belonging to either one. Whenever I went back home to visit, I was a visitor, an outsider. I've lived in my adopted home of California for more than thirty-five years, yet I'll always be an immigrant. In a way, I was perpetually on a search for a place where I felt truly at home.

It still amazed me that I could call my mother across the ocean while sitting on a rock in a campground a world away. I didn't have to collect a fistful of quarters, try to dial an international operator while praying my parents would be home and then rushing to say as much as possible before I got cut off in the middle of the sentence when the last quarter dropped. When I first arrived in the States back in the eighties, a phone call was a luxury I could only afford every so often. I would be so nervous and excited to hear my parents over the phone that I'd get diarrhea. Airmail letters were our main form of communication. Each letter was so special, and I awaited it with great anticipation. I would read them over and over and pin them on the walls of every room I ever rented, so I was surrounded by the words of my family. That's how I created my sanctuary.

I still have stacks of those letters.

Many include recipes from my mother, grandmother, sister-in-law, and cousins. I learned to cook through family letters. Growing up, our main meals always started with clear beef or chicken bone broth soup with homemade fine egg noodles Grandma Hani and Grandpa Joško made. After my grandpa suffered a stroke, kneading, rolling and cutting the pasta dough was his therapy. The soup was not complicated, but I had to ask my mother for her exact recipe. When I was young, I'd been too impatient to learn.

After I left home and was so far away and feeling homesick and lonely, I began to understand how food connects people. Once in the States, I would learn through letters how many carrots, garlic cloves, onions, how much parsley, pepper and salt to add along with the soup bones and exactly how long to cook it. My kids, who call my mother Babi, now ask me, "How do you make Babi soup? How do you make Babi chicken? Babi potatoes?"

When I first learned to cook the food of my homeland, I'd stick to less complicated dishes like angel pee pees, which are potato dough dumplings sprinkled with breadcrumbs and sautéed in butter. It might have been my kids and their friends' favorite food just because they could giggle saying *Angel Pee Pees* out loud.

My grandmother had a sister who left our war-torn country after World War II. I was very fond of my great-aunt Ladi. After she died, her daughters gave me a stack of letters that were written in Slovene. One letter, written on a very thin, almost transparent paper, detailed the proper way to butcher a pig and make sausages. It included detailed instructions on making use of every part of the animal. I am quite certain I will never try to make my own blood sausages. After Ladi and her husband, Josef, emigrated, her mother-in-law sent the instructions:

Cool the butchered meat. Salt the meat and let it sit over-night. The next day boil salted water—not too much salt—let the water cool down and submerge meat entirely in it. Then sauté meat in hot oil and fat but not so hot as to not burn the meat. Make sure all meat is sautéed or it will become moldy. I watched Zofka do that; now I do the same, and it works. The meat is very tasty this way. To make sausages, cook rice but not too soft. Add quite a bit of onion to oil. Onion needs to become yellow, add pepper, marjoram and a little blood. Do not boil blood for more than ten minutes. Then cool the meat off, stuff the sausage casings, and then you can bake them again and you will now have European food to eat. I am attaching two photos of us so your daughters will see how Opapa and Omama look. We are already very old and ugly now. The photographs are not as you would have made them, Josef, but they were taken because we needed new documents now that we have a new country.

Emails and all the new technologies have changed our form of communication so much. Will we be able to retrieve and keep some of our communication for future generations?

It does make me nostalgic for receiving a real letter or a postcard that I can touch and smell. My favorite ones contained dried alpine flowers pressed by my mother. I would carefully cut the letter open with a knife to preserve the envelope. I also wanted to prolong the satisfaction before reading what my mother, my father, and sometimes even my brother wrote. I would first inhale the opened envelope. Out would slip a violet gentian wildflower. The smell of the flower would immediately transport me back home in my mind, and I could smell the mountains and the high alpine fields. Limestone baking in the sun, the grasses, and the earth after the rains and the lush and damp forests were the smells that I would miss for the longest time after I left my home. I still miss those aromas—those places.

After the call to my mother, I returned to the endless project of assessing my gear.

I turned on my Garmin, only to find that the new map from Lake Isabella to the border had magically disappeared. What the hell? I had a backup on my iPhone, but I hadn't figured out how to transfer it without my laptop. Cruel joke! *Is this a test, or is it a message?* I wondered.

Dealing with technology was one of my biggest challenges. Just when I thought I had things figured out, something else would happen. I wanted to hurl the GPS unit against a boulder. I should have practiced more before I left home. I was overly confident that things were just going to work out. I still had some time before crossing the border to figure it out, and I had to because once I crossed into Mexico, I'd be in a lot more rugged and remote terrain, and proper navigation would be crucial. I would need to be resolute, vigilant, and resilient. When I was dealing with serious medical issues, it was hard to think of myself as resilient. I now had a chance to rekindle that dormant spirit.

While climbing the steep hills, I was reminded again of my roots. As a tiny nation, Slovenia always had to fight for its existence. During World War II, our region was occupied by the Italians before Hitler marched into the city of Maribor on April 26, 1941, declaring, "Machen Sie mir dieses Land wieder deutsch!" (Make this land German for me again!) Burning two and a half million books written in Slovene and shipping intellectuals to concentration camps by the trainload was an attempt to eliminate the entire nation. As a young boy in first grade, my father was part of the resistance. Under the guidance of their teacher, he and his classmates helped smuggle Slovenian books into a hidden cellar just before the Germans burned the library. He showed his resilient spirit at a young age. When the going got tough, I had to remind myself I was my father's daughter, fighting for my own existence.

There would be fewer chances to opt out the farther south I went.

I heated up a three-day-old egg burrito, managed to burn it to a near-charcoaled state, and packed up my gear, slowly and methodically. I called it packing meditation. I couldn't find my one and only bra. Plus, I was still using a fork for a comb. I hadn't been able to find a place that would sell just one stupid comb. Everything was in a pack of three or more. As I was ruminating on commercial excess, the bra revealed itself under my Thermarest. I still found it difficult to comprehend how much gear I could pack on the bike. I laid everything on a picnic table and stared at it. Was there anything I could live without?

I had already made a big mistake sending my warm gear home before I should have. Now I was feeling afraid to part with anything. I could find a reason for every item and was sure my life would depend on it. In the town of Lake Isabella, I stopped to have a proper cup of coffee and a breakfast sandwich and to get Wi-Fi so I could deal with loading the route I was missing. After an hour with Lee from Garmin tech support, we finally paired my phone and Edge 1030 and managed to load the missing map. He was very patient with me. My mood lifted, and I took off following the purple line. My Garmin, strapped on my handlebar, started beeping that I was off course while prompting me to make a U-turn.

What the heck? I looked at the map again, and it was stuck in the direction from south to north. Defeated again, I sat in the park under a tree. It was eighty degrees and rising. I tried unsuccessfully to load the new map. Then I tried rotating the map I had. No such luck! I decided, the hell with it! I rode following the map backward. It worked, but everything was in reverse, and Garmin kept beeping annoyingly, prompting me to turn around to ride north toward home. I was tempted.

I climbed out of the Kern Valley, leaving Lake Isabella behind. The wind was at my back as two red-tailed hawks circled, looking for their daily meal. I was in a completely different environment: high, dry desert. After climbing and dropping over two more passes and riding through the historic town of Havilah, I zigzagged back and forth on a steep road toward what I thought was a general store or restaurant. I was disappointed. It was just a fenced-off house with a giant American flag flying over it. I stopped to take a picture when a ferocious pit bull came barreling around the corner. The thick chain stopped her massive square head just before she reached the fence in a plume of dust, which matched the color of her shiny gray coat. I was only inches away from the dog's frothing, angry, spit-flying jaws. Holy crap! My heart was in my throat, and I scrambled on The Beast and took off. This was not a friendly place. I flew downhill with the dog barking after me for a long, long time.

Across the flats, I battled some strong headwinds, so when I reached the base of the next climb, I pulled over at a corral with two miniature horses and some baby cows. I had a shot of GU, which is uber-sweet energy food with the consistency of cake frosting, and some water, which was beginning to run low.

A car pulled up to the house across the road. Out stepped a young woman. I heard her speaking Spanish to someone inside. I ran across with my water bottle and asked for some water. The young girl didn't speak much English, but she said, "Yes, yes, water, *agua*, no problem!"

I switched to Spanish, and while she went into the house for water,

I met her father who worked for the rancher. The ranch had fifty horses and they offered guided multiday tours into the mountains. The father, an experienced Mexican vaquero, took care of all the horses. His daughter Estrella came out with three bottles of water while her mother called out to ask me if I wanted a taco for the road.

"*Por supuesto que sí! Gracias, señora!*" I said gratefully. That would be very nice, thank you!

In the meantime, while the mother was preparing food inside, Estrella and I chatted. She'd just had a baby six weeks earlier. I told her where I was going, what I ate, where I slept. I said that I was riding to Mexico. She told me her family was from Michoacán. Her baby daughter's name was Amber.

I went back across the street to put the water on my bike. She followed me with a grilled ham and cheese sandwich and a bag of fruit. I tried to explain that I didn't have much room on my bike, but I couldn't refuse such generosity. I tied the plastic bag onto the back, adding yet another bulky accessory to my already overloaded Beast. Then the mother came with another bag full of snacks. I tried again to tell them there's no more room, but they insisted. Totally charmed and moved by their hospitality and kindness, I was able to stuff two hot slices of pizza, something wrapped in a heavy white piece of paper, a cup of instant soup, string cheese, yogurt, and some snacks I've never even seen before, into every nook and cranny on The Beast. I hugged the two women and wished them the happiest of lives. I didn't know if I'd ever be able to repay them, but I could certainly pay it forward. They waved me off with wishes of safe travels. I was so filled with gratitude that I flew up the hill.

I'd only made it a few hundred yards before I had to stop again. Overcome with emotion, I put my head on the handlebars and cried. These are hardworking people, family-loving people who clean and cook and build and run this country quietly, behind the scenes. This country was built and is continuing to be built on the shoulders of immigrants from all over the world, including Estrella's family and me. I worked my way through college taking every job I could find, from sandblasting sailboat masts to painting houses to busing tables in roadside diners.

It took me a long time to pull myself together. As it got late, I looked for places to pitch my tent. I had a signal, so I talked to Jim on the phone as I rode.

"It looks like Caliente is just five miles away and downhill," he informed me.

I pictured a cute town with a tavern, cold beer, and a hot meal, and I was sure there would be a campground.

I literally rode into the sunset as I crested over the last hill. The sun set behind the clouds, outlining them in bright orange like a Renaissance painting. I pictured Raphael's fat cherubs with bows and arrows.

Caliente was just around the corner. I loved riding the steep down-hill until I came around a corner and almost crashed into a herd of cattle crossing the road. I slammed on the brakes. They stared at me, not moving. My headlamp reflected in their eyes, making them shine bright red. They looked possessed, black as night. I started moving slowly, observing how they would react.

"Good cow, good cow, stay where you are!" I told them.

I talked to them in a calming voice, hoping my red jacket wouldn't excite them. Two cows, a mom and not-so-small calf separated by the road, started running. I kept riding slowly, hoping they'd stop and get away from the road, away from me. There was a turn up ahead, and a car was coming fast in the opposite direction. I was sure the car was going to hit one of the running cows. The brakes squealed, and the car came to a skidding stop inches away from the calf. I rode slowly by as a rancher on a quad came to corral the cattle into a gated pasture.

Twilight. The time of the evening when bats dart in all directions, feeding on insects and pollinating a variety of flowers, some of which only bloom at night. Since their echolocation system is precise, I never worried they'd ever run into me, but sometimes they darted only inches from my head, and I ducked instinctively. The first sliver of the moon played peek-a-boo from behind the hills. I should have been in Caliente already. I kept riding but came upon nothing. It was now completely dark, and my track was taking me on a quiet, lonely country road away from Caliente. What was going on? Jim was calling me, and of course, he was concerned, as was I. As he was following me on the maps on his iPhone, he could see my dot moving away from Caliente.

"There was no town anywhere! Not a house in sight!" I told him.

"How's that possible?" Caliente shows up on the map, I am looking at it!"

"I can't figure it out! It's dark. I have to find a place to camp. I'll call you back when I do!" I was looking for places to pitch the tent, but I knew that Jim would worry and wouldn't sleep if I was camped on the side of a lonely country road. Thinking of snakes, I wasn't excited about setting up a tent in the dark in tall dry grass. I kept riding, climbing for another thousand vertical feet until the track took me onto Highway 58. Huge semis flew by me. I was on the phone with Jim, his daughter, Jenna, and her husband, Brett, and they were looking at the maps at home.

"The closest possible stop is the town of Keene, which is still another ten miles away!" They told me when they called back.

"Okay great! No worries, I got this. It's easy riding, and the road is wide and safe," I lied to Jim.

No big deal in a car, but a big deal on a bike at night with semis roaring by. I hated it. The plastic bag full of fruit was banging against the rear wheel, and it split open, sending plums and apples flying onto the road, where the passing truck ran them over. *This might soon be me*, I thought as I watched an apple roll under the wheel of a semi. The road kept climbing. I was weary, but finally reached Keene, which consisted of a coffee shop and a fire station with a helicopter port next to it.

I almost fell off the bike at nine thirty that night and was forced by darkness to set up the tent under a large tree behind the closed coffee shop. I changed my sweaty clothes, climbed into my sleeping bag, and unwrapped the white paper Estrella's mother gave me. It was half a breast of fried chicken, the best damn chicken I'd ever eaten in my life! For dessert, I ate a juicy-sweet poached pear she gave me that I'd carried all the way in a plastic cup on the back of my bike. Tears of exhaustion and gratitude flew down my cheeks as I tried to get comfortable. I dozed off but was soon startled by some people talking and casting shadows toward my tent by walking in front of their car lights, the car engine running. I held my breath and listened. Can they see my tent? Did I lock up my bike? It's past eleven o'clock! What are they doing out here at this late hour?

Then the doors slammed, and the car took off. I was jacked up on adrenaline but so exhausted that I drifted off into a semiconscious state of sleep. The whole night, it felt like the trucks going by on the freeway and the nearby trains were coming right through the tent. Every time I heard a car, my head popped up and I thought, *They're back*!

I was thrilled when the Keene Coffee Shop opened at seven.

Fifty-three miles, 5,600 feet of climbing, and more than ten hours in the saddle made for a long day. I had been challenged every day of my ride. I was questioning my abilities in the most demanding of moments while exhausted to the bone. Then, somehow, lying in my tent at night resting, I was able to remind myself why I was doing all this. Somehow, by the time the sun rose, I found the will to continue. Every moment like that was a triumph. I was living life to the hilt, feeling exhilarated and grateful. I only wished I could have shared the agony and the ecstasy with those I loved.

—THIRTEEN—
Si, Se Puede!

It doesn't take much to make me happy;
You know now that ordinary warm water in the faucet
will do the trick.
—Isabel Allende

It was Thursday, October 11, and I was the first customer at the Keene Coffee Shop. Over breakfast, I considered my progress. Now that I had checked off one map and started following a new one, I realized I had ridden 611 miles and climbed more than 57,300 vertical feet riding twelve days straight. Without a doubt, this was the longest and the farthest I had ever ridden in my life. I felt proud.

While enjoying breakfast and hot coffee, I was reading about the history of the coffee shop on the back of the menu. It used to serve as a boarding house for limestone miners back in the late 1800s and saw its heyday during World War II when it was a hangout for soldiers who were guarding nearby railroad tunnels.

I took a washcloth into the bathroom and cleaned with scalding hot water. I was stark naked, so I kept checking the door to make sure it was locked. A hot shower is such a small luxury in life. It's hard to believe a woman of my age would be washing herself in a roadside café bathroom. But I was doing it for fun, not out of necessity like so many homeless people all over the world are forced to do.

After my wash-up and morning meal, I climbed out of Keene on the Tehachapi Loop, passing the national monument of Cesar Chavez at the National Chavez Center. SI SE PUEDE! read the sign I passed. Yes, we can! The rallying cry and motto of the United Farm Workers of America since 1972.

Even though the road was climbing, it was pleasantly winding away from Highway 58. I passed small, neatly kept farmhouses with antique trucks out front. It was like riding through a living museum. When I reached the crest, I stopped and took in the view of the Tehachapi railroad loop, one of the Seven Wonders of the World's railroads. It was built between 1874 and 1876 by mostly Chinese laborers from Canton, now a Guangdong Province.

I coasted into the town of Tehachapi just after noon and went to SaveMart to get some blueberries and to look for that ever-elusive comb. Damn multipacks! Out of principle, I still refused to buy them.

I crossed the Mojave Desert, riding into hot winds and through the town of Lancaster, passing Jack In The Box, McDonald's, Denny's, Burger King, Taco Bell, and Kentucky Fried Chicken. I turned the corner onto another street, and they repeated, just not in the same order. After passing KFC at the end of the second block, I felt nauseated from the smell of frying oil.

One of the things that most frustrated me about my cancer was trying to figure out how and why I got it. There is medical evidence that sugar, fat, and processed foods contribute greatly. I shop at farmers' markets and cook from scratch. It didn't seem fair. Of course, there are many factors that significantly contribute to developing breast cancer. Most of those listed in medical journals and studies didn't apply to me. I always ate healthy foods, drank in moderation, exercised regularly, and most importantly, had no genetic predisposition. None of my family members have ever had breast cancer. But there was one factor that made me wonder. Stress. Several studies, including one Swedish study, suggest that stress, especially severe stress like divorce or the death of a child, can put a person at much higher risk, just like smoking puts you at higher risk of lung cancer or heart disease. I've been told I appear tough and capable of dealing with issues. In truth, I have always held my deepest emotions close to my heart. My stresses piled up. I suffered a devastating blow in the years leading up to my divorce. The stress continued to build during our process of uncoupling and for years after the divorce. In the end it got so bad I couldn't enter the house after I'd return from a long business trip. I'd round the last corner to our house and slow the car to a crawl; then I'd just sit in it for hours, even if it was the middle of the night. My kids were asleep in their beds. I was outside in the driveway. I wanted to hold them but couldn't cross the threshold.

I rode to the outskirts of Lancaster toward Palmdale, blasted by a prevailing east wind so strong, I had to lean into it so I wouldn't get knocked over. I rode past numerous pawn shops, used car dealerships, and rundown motels with young women dressed in skimpy clothes on phones working to get clients, desperate to make some money. Whenever I'd see that, I'd think of my own daughters and how much I had worried for their future.

I couldn't wait to get out of town, but that, too, was the part of the landscape I was riding through. I followed the Garmin's purple line as the San Gabriel Mountains rose before me. Few canyons lead into them. I wondered which one was going to take me up and through. I got lost, rode an extra ten miles up the steep hill, but then a smooth downhill with a bit of a tailwind, and The Beast and I set a new speed record: 39.57 mph—damn, so close to hitting forty! That was pretty fast on a loaded mountain bike with fat tires. As I flew down the hill, the old feeling I would rarely achieve during a downhill ski race returned. In coaching, we referred to that as being in the zone. I was relaxed. I had an easy smile on my face, I was breathing through my nose, and I was in complete control and aware of my surroundings. I was flying, but it appeared as if everything else around me were moving in slow motion. I could feel the wind on my face as I leaned forward, scooped low with my shoulders, my elbows tucked in and hidden behind the bags on the front of my handlebars. I rose slightly and moved behind the saddle as far as the attached bags allowed me to, so I could arch my back to have the least possible amount of air resistance. I pressed my knees against the frame of my bike as if I were squeezing the belly of a horse really tight, giving it direction. The Beast and I became one. We were moving at our greatest possible speed at that moment. The time-space continuum ceased to exist for a few seemingly endless moments. It was as if I were being sucked into an invisible tunnel. Once again, I was a speed demon, racing on my bike instead of racing on skis. Oh, the pure joy of it! Up we went for another several miles to yet another summit, and then coasted into the camp of Monte Cristo at an elevation of 3,600 feet. I rode around, but all the campsites were filled with guys in camouflage hunting gear.

I found what I thought was an empty site and set up my tent. A slim guy who was raking his campsite across the road kept looking at me, and not in a friendly way. When I was all set up and ready to go pay, I stopped to chat with my neighbor, who, it turned out, was the camp host.

"All campsites have been reserved for months in advance," he said. "Tomorrow is the start of hunting season."

The slim guy walked over and introduced himself as Ming. He

informed me I was on his site, pointing to the tiny white tag on the post of "my" campsite.

"Well, jeez, Ming, why didn't you say something while I was setting up?"

He didn't answer. Instead, he told me that his boss was on his way. So were many other people. He kept raking around me. "Wives, kids, dogs, lots of people! Lots of noise!"

The camp host, an old Vietnam vet with a long gray ponytail and a red bandanna holding his thinning gray hair, walked up and said to Ming, "Look, you guys have three campsites. She doesn't take up much room. Let her stay and share this site."

Ming was nice enough, and he said, "Okay, no problem; you can stay."

"Should I move my tent?"

"Oh no, it's okay."

He went across to his other site, and cars started pulling in. Coolers, stoves, tables, chairs, and lamps came out. They made fires, tossed steaks on the grill, and it smelled so good. I suddenly realized I was starving. I started the battle with my stove to heat a cup of instant chicken noodle soup, and I popped open a can of tuna that I scooped out with crumbled jalapeño chips. Delicious! But the smell of grilled steak next door was making me dizzy. It was now eight o'clock and dark, so I brushed my teeth and crawled into my tent. I dozed off despite my neighbors' generators, music, and laughter.

"Ma'am? Ma'am!"

"Yes," I replied in a groggy voice.

"Ma'am, you are quite close to the fire pit, and these guys are going to have a fire." I realized the voice belonged to Steve, the camp host.

Indeed, another group had just pulled in and were setting up their tents and bringing out all their gear. I pulled out the tent stakes and dragged my tent away. Then I introduced myself, thanked them for letting me share their site, and went back to bed. They weren't very friendly, and I didn't blame them. I was in their space. While I was dragging the tent, I forgot I had a cup of cocoa inside and as I dragged it over, it spilled. Sticky sweet liquid now covered my pad and sleeping bag. I got my micro towel and wiped it off as best I could and fell back onto my two-inch-thick Thermarest. I tossed and turned trying to get comfortable again. It was a long night of generators roaring, car doors slamming, dogs barking, and kids screaming. I stuffed some rolled-up toilet paper in my ears and somehow drifted into dreamland.

I woke up in the middle of the night. The parties had finally died down, but it was raining. The raindrops on the tent lulled me back to sleep. I woke up again at five to slamming doors and cars taking off all around me. The hunters. Oh, there is going to be blood today! I closed my eyes, and the face of a dead deer stared at me with her big black moist eyes. I couldn't get rid of the image.

I packed up my soaking gear early in the morning while it was still raining and headed into the San Gabriel Mountains. As I climbed the remote Upper Big Tujunga Road, the smells after the rain were intense and new to me. The flora of this area was unfamiliar yet deeply intoxicating. It seemed I was able to inhale a full deep breath for the first time since my cancer diagnosis. I climbed toward a 7,000-foot summit enshrouded in thick fog. I turned on my lights on the helmet and the back of the bike so drivers could see me. Birds sang, and I heard gunshots from hunters. It suddenly occurred to me that I could be mistaken for a deer. As this thought crossed my mind, two deer crossed the road in front of me.

As I was gaining elevation and the air was cooling off, my right leg started cramping. It was clear that the nerve damage I'd suffered during knee surgery manifested even more at high altitude and lower temperatures. It had been more than two years since the surgery, and there'd been no improvement. The muscles in my back and my glutes seized up. I had to get off my bike frequently to shake and massage the muscles loose again. It was a pattern on every climb. It was not something that I was by any means getting used to.

I was told back at the Monte Cristo campground that there was a restaurant called Newcomb's Ranch on the way to the next campsite, about twenty-seven miles away. Good news, as I was out of food. It was a long day of climbing over 4,000 vertical feet. And there it was, a lovely mountain lodge! I was salivating.

I got off the bike and walked to the door with a skip in my step. I pulled the handle of a heavy wooden door, which didn't budge. I pulled harder. Nothing! Then I noticed a yellow note tacked on the door, right in my face. "Sorry, we had to close today due to problems with our sewer system."

I rattled the door and screamed, "Why? Why in bloody hell can I not get a fucking break! What have I done to be tested and punished all the time! I just want some goddamn food!" I sat down next to my bike. I spat out cursing words worse than my husband when he was fixing his broken machines in the garage. It was like everything I've been holding inside of me for the last few years came vomiting out. I looked around, terrified by my outburst. Oh, my god! I hoped no one had seen me as I wiped spit off my chin, embarrassed.

It was such a letdown after my built-up anticipation. That always happens whenever I have expectations that are not met: a deep, gut-wrenching disappointment. I told myself I needed to work on that; that it's better not to have expectations. But the words rang hollow in my empty belly and just made me feel grumpier.

As I sat there, a couple approached and told me that they had driven from Hollywood and were equally crushed, but obviously not displaying such an outburst. The woman, whose name was Sisi, said, "Look, someone is sitting at the bar inside. Let's walk to the back door and see if it's open!"

I reluctantly pushed the door ajar and called into a darkened space. A soccer game resounded in Spanish from a large TV screen in the corner.

"Hello, anyone here?"

A small Mexican guy named Sam came around the corner.

"Sorry, closed!"

"Yes, I know; can I just buy some snacks?"

Sisi came behind me and explained to him in rapid Spanish that I was on a long ride to Mexico.

"I'll go ask the boss," said Sam, who was the cook at the restaurant. After a while, he came out with an egg and avocado sandwich on sourdough bread and ham and lettuce on an English muffin. I was again overcome with gratitude, and as I was finishing my egg and avocado sandwich, Sam brought me a bottle of water and a Snapple. I handed him a twenty-dollar bill, but he refused to take it. I literally forced the bill into his pocket.

"People are so amazing!" I said to Sisi. "The less they have, the more generous they are!" I told her about my Mexican family experience and how they had gifted me all that food. She asked what the hardest part of my trip had been so far. I told her about all the big climbs and the freezing nights. She told me she couldn't imagine. She'd never slept in a tent before. I told her I was pining for the warmth of Mexico.

"Wait," she said. "I got something for you."

She walked toward the car, where her boyfriend had been sitting the whole time, never getting out. I think he was really pissed about the restaurant being closed. She came back and handed me a long, heavy black wool coat.

I thanked her but said there's no way I could take it. She tried to assure me it was okay— that she has plenty of coats back home. I told her she was so kind, and I wished I could take it. I really did. But I had no room, and I couldn't ride in a coat that heavy and big.

"Okay, I understand," she said. "But I hate it that you are so cold."

I told her that her generosity would keep me warm at night. We hugged, and they drove off back to Hollywood in their Mustang. I finished my sandwich and tucked away my English muffin for dinner.

After a few more miles riding on the Ángeles Crest Highway, I reached a campground nestled on a hill among redwoods and boulders. It was five o'clock on Saturday, and I quickly realized that all the sites were full again. A young girl came out of the bathroom, and we started talking.

"Oh, you can camp at our site. There's plenty of room."

I thanked her profusely as I was tired and just wanted to get off my bike and set up the tent for the night. We were at 6,500 feet, and it was cooling off fast. My tent and all my gear were still soaked from the previous night's rain.

I heated up some water for a cup of miso soup and ate the rest of my food from the diner. The young group I was sharing the campsite with was playing beer pong. Their two unruly dogs barked incessantly. I could already see I'd made a big mistake, but my camp was set up.

Just down the hill, there was a community fire. I headed down, and I met four families with young kids running around and roasting marshmallows. We connected instantly. A French–German couple with a three-year-old trilingual daughter, Leah, invited me to move to their camp.

"Aw, that's okay, thank you! It's too much work to move everything. Quiet time is at ten anyway."

We sat around and talked and ate marshmallows. The kids fell asleep in their parents' arms, one by one with sticky fingers and dirty faces. My mind flooded with memories of many a campfire with my kids when they were little. I wanted to borrow one of the little ones and snuggle. I missed my children so much it hurt. At around nine, I crawled into my damp tent and damp sleeping bag. I was dressed in three jackets, long underwear, and sweatpants, each layer saturated and damp. I wore my fleece hat my friend Emily had made over the hood of my merino wool shirt. I looked as if I were preparing to camp on Mt. Everest. It was already thirty-seven degrees. The sky was clear, so I knew the temperature would drop. It went to thirty degrees by morning. I've climbed mountains in winter, ski raced, and ski coached, but I don't think I've ever been so cold in my life. I was sure it was amplified by how tired I was. I wished I'd brought a warmer sleeping bag. Then I wished I had accepted Sisi's big, heavy coat. And the beer pong? It went on at least until midnight! I stopped checking the time, but since they allowed me to share a site with them, I felt it wasn't my place to tell them to quiet down. Oh, how I wanted to.

In the morning, I struggled with my stove to heat up water for tea and my last bag of oatmeal. The fire was already going at the family camp, so I headed down. What a welcome heat after a freezing night. Pretty soon, Dan, one of the dads, handed me a full plate of scrambled eggs and bacon, and his two adorable kids, Ryder and Jolene, made pancakes in a large cast-iron skillet over the fire. My heart and my stomach were full, and my body was slowly thawing. Soon, the rest of the families joined, and Dan fed everyone.

As I rode away toward Wrightwood, I thought of how many

interesting, kind, and generous people I'd already met. The water givers, the food sharers, the fist pumpers, the thumbs-ups, and the "You go, girl!" hollers. The places I rode through were amazingly beautiful. The sweeping vistas of the peaks protruding above the clouds, endless golden hills studded with giant granite boulders with cows as black as night grazing lazily among them. Thick, dark virgin forests with streaks of light protruding through the thick canopy, lighting up remote and lonely roads for me and showing me the way like a beacon of hope. It was the people who were painting my memories in bright colors.

I really can catch a break, I told myself. Every time I am met with misfortune, a person walks into my life and shines light on me with their love, kindness, and generosity. I am still here, living my dream, aren't I? I entered a tunnel on the road and was again swallowed up by the darkness. With everything disappearing around me, I thought of my angry, embarrassing overreaction when I arrived at the closed restaurant. Then Sam made me a sandwich, and Sisi offered me her warm coat. It was a simple act of giving that changed everything. That anger bursting out of me with such fury had much deeper origins.

It was poisoning me. It scared me.

I didn't want to be that angry person. I could see the light at the end of the tunnel and rode into it, feeling another layer of darkness peeling away.

—FOURTEEN—
The Devil Winds

Need to put footsteps of courage into the stirrup of patience.
—Ernest Shackleton

I climbed for about 2,400 feet and stopped at the Grassy Hollow ranger station where the Pacific Crest Trail crosses the road. I had a friendly chat and an instant connection with Ranger Joanne, also a breast cancer survivor. She used to be a high-powered executive in the City of Angels. After cancer, she found her happiness in the mountains. She was done with the hustle and bustle of the big concrete jungle, left a high-paying job, and decided to become a ranger. What inspiration! It takes guts to do that! To leave everything behind and start fresh. I felt I'd found a kindred spirit. Joanne gave me some helpful information about the next town. I looked forward to a much-needed rest for the afternoon. I was excited to sleep in a warm, comfortable bed—and perhaps I'd find a comb. My hair was getting tangled and knotted under the helmet, and it hadn't been properly combed since I'd left home. I considered the possibility of forgetting all about finding a comb and instead just growing dreadlocks. It felt good to laugh.

I arrived in Wrightwood in midafternoon, just after passing another ski area. I'd been a skier all my life and lived in a ski resort

town in Northern California, and I didn't know they had so many
ski areas in Southern California, the land of endless surf beaches. I
began my routine of looking for a place to spend the night. I needed
to dry my gear, so I decided to stay at Cedar Lodge in the middle of
this cute resort town. The room was large, and I hung my wet clothing and camping gear on every wall hook and piece of furniture. The
large screen TV was draped in my tent fly, pink underwear adorned
the lampshade on the right side of the bed, and my one and only gray
sports bra on the left. I took a long hot shower, which I'd longed for,
combed my hair with a fork, and walked across the street to a bar.
Oktoberfest was in full swing with decorations, music, a five-dollar
traditional German dinner, and good German Spaten beer. The beer
made me sleepy, so I returned to the safety and comfort of my room.

The next morning, I walked to a coffee shop where a few older
men sat on the deck in the sun, warming up like old cats. I pushed
open the door, and the lady asked, "You need a haircut, dear?"

"Oh, no, thanks! Just some breakfast."

"The coffee shop is next door, but it's closed on Mondays," she
replied. I realized I'd entered the wrong door. I began to apologize
and retreated, but then paused. It was my rest day. Might as well get
pampered a bit.

"Wait, do you have time for a haircut?"

"Sure, girl. Come on in," said the woman, whose name was Heidi,
happy to get an unexpected customer.

I was so tempted to cut my hair super short! Vanity got the better
of me, and I chickened out. I thought of Jim's comment from those
years back when he didn't like my hair short. I did care, maybe more
than ever, about how Jim saw me. My hair was still growing out after
I'd been bald for such a long time. I thought about how painful it had
been for Jim to watch me being so sick and bald. He'd suffered quietly,

as was his way. Besides, I could finally make a tiny little ponytail. I decided to just get a trim and some highlights, to brighten things up a bit.

And I finally got a comb, compliments of my new favorite stylist. My days of fork-combing were over.

I was planning to stay for a day of rest, but Heidi told me that the ride to Crestline was mostly downhill and not that far, just an easy climb "and then you'll be home free," she promised.

I hurried back to my room, quickly packed up all my stuff, and was back on the road. Just before I left town, I went to the hardware store, and a very nice lady named Davon helped me change the batteries for the light on the back of my helmet. As she did, we chatted about all kinds of things. I was struck by her kindness, and Heidi's too. I asked her if everyone in town drank some kind of special juice that made them so nice. She laughed.

"We drink all right, but the juice sure is not it, Honey." I'd been called "Honey" an awful lot on this trip.

I headed out of town. It was windy and cold, but I looked forward to a day without too much climbing. After all, Heidi, the hairdresser, said so.

Eventually, The Beast and I reached Silverwood Lake. Eleven miles to go to reach Crestline. We got this. No big deal! The yellow sign warned there were sharp turns ahead: TRUCKS USE CAUTION. Oh, this is going to be a fun downhill! And then the road started climbing. I mean rising at a 10 percent grade! I kept chanting mantras to myself: "Don't get off the bike, don't get off the bike!" and "Everything has to end, everything has to end." I barely hung on, crawling in my lowest gear at a snail's pace. I had to pull over every few turns to catch my breath. I decided that was the last time I would listen to a hairdresser.

I reached Crestline entirely spent. I rolled into town, which was trying to look cute with imitation Bavarian architecture. Seemed to be a common appearance, immigrants attempting to recreate their home country's architecture, but the imitation never looked quite right. Sleepy Hollow had cabins and rooms. I got a special deal on a room used for storage with a pullout couch for a bed. Anything that was cheap and warm would do. The best thing about the motel was that it had an outdoor Jacuzzi. As soon as I carried my bike up the stairs with the help of the manager, I changed into my shorts and headed back downstairs. Strong jets massaged my sore muscles, and I slowly recovered. I had the Jacuzzi all to myself, which was a good thing, as I was sitting in my one and only sports bra and my only pair of underwear (There was no room on my bike for a bathing suit.). It was a great opportunity to do laundry at the same time.

Famished, I headed down the street to Tony's Mexican restaurant. I ordered a double combo, and the oval shape plate that the waitress held with both hands took over half the table. It was overflowing with beans, rice, two chimichangas, and a chile relleno. My eyes popped wide, convinced I couldn't eat all of it. But I did. All of it without any guilt because I'd been burning more calories than I could replace. I washed the food down with a Corona, and I was ready to pass out. I burped and farted all the way back to my room, fell into the lumpy couch bed, and was soon gone to dreamland.

My dream was vivid. I'm flying one of those glider two-seater ultra-light planes. Behind me sits my friend Doug. We fly from Stanford Medical Center up to Tahoe for a day after I kidnap him from the hospital. First, we fly just over the tops of the city skyscrapers, and then over the mountains. Somehow, I maneuver under a bunch of electric wires and under the Old Donner Pass Bridge. "We're almost home!" I yell at Doug. We both wear leather helmets and round classic aviation goggles. It's a crazy and dangerous flight, but I navigate expertly. We laugh. Doug is happy because he can escape the hospital and go home, even if it's just for a day. I am happy I can fly with him.

In the morning, I remembered the dream so vividly, which doesn't always happen. I wished I had a plane and I wished I could fly Doug to Tahoe. Instead, I had to just fly with him in my mind on the wings of my bike, wondering about the meaning of the dream. I definitely was not alone in this fight with cancer. Doug had been at Stanford Hospital undergoing a stem cell transplant for myelofibrosis, a rare type of cancer in which the bone marrow is replaced by fibrous scar tissue. It is considered a form of chronic leukemia. Doug and his wife Laura were on a long and arduous ride. They had been at the hospital for months. Doug had been diagnosed just a few months after he shaved my head. I thought of them so often during my journey. Doug has such a positive outlook on life. I had no doubt he was going to pull through, but he had to get through this part of his difficult journey first. His pain was my pain.

As I climbed into the whipping Santa Ana headwinds, I unclipped my pedals just in time to catch myself from falling over. There was no shoulder on the Rim of the World Highway. It was hard to enjoy the spectacular view across the valley from the San Bernardino Mountains. I hated every meter of that downright deadly ride. The wind made me cranky. Good thing no one was riding with me or I'd have bitten their head off. Big Bear Lake still seemed so far away. The winds were not just mercilessly strong but had an edge of winter in them. They call them the Devil Winds for a good reason. The peaks around me were covered with snow. I finally reached the top of the climb at 7,000 feet. Big Bear Lake lay in the distance. I couldn't wait to get the ride over for the day. My hands and feet were stiff and cold. My rear wheel had started to make an annoying clicking sound. I tried to ignore it. If you ignore something, it'll just go away, right?

Well, it didn't. I pulled over and climbed off the bike, always a balancing act. I spun the rear wheel slowly with my right hand, while holding my heavy bike off the ground with my left. And there it was: a thorn in my tire. I pulled it out and with it came a "hiss" of air as white slime oozed out of the tube. Not good. Not good at all! Then I remembered what Carl and Wane at Olympic Bike taught me, "Spin the wheel as fast as you can!" It worked! The slime inside the tire sealed the hole all on its own. I pulled out the pump to add air. The valve on the tire was bent, so every time I tried to attach the pump, more air escaped. If I broke the valve, I was screwed! Since I only had about five miles more to go, I decided to continue limping to Big Bear on a flat tire. I found it difficult to appreciate my beautiful surroundings because I was so tired, hungry, and cold. Big Bear Lake was very much reminiscent of Lake Tahoe. I looked for a campground, but the idea of setting up a tent and freezing all night again wasn't appealing. Just down the road, there was a Travelodge. The forty-five-dollar price was right. The guy at the desk was missing a few teeth but was very friendly and honored a AAA discount, even though I didn't have my card with me. Once I got to my room, a hot bath, instant hot soup, and a cup of cocoa warmed me. I'd never anticipated riding in such cold weather and climbing such challenging hills through Southern California. Ignorance sure is bliss, and perhaps so is not having the ability or the inclination to plan ahead. Had I known, would I have gone? One doesn't see into the future for a good reason.

I was on a quest seeking balance. On one end was freedom of the road and the wide-open spaces, on the other the security and familiarity of home. Bathing in solitude, riding on remote roads, I finally felt like I was in charge of my own destiny and not being controlled and dictated by doctor appointments and painful treatments. I could make my own decisions about everything between sunrise and sunset, often until the moon chased me down. Shining brightly on me, the moon helped me set up my tent at night. I only needed to prove myself to myself out there. With every laborious deep breath I took, the air that was sucked out of every crevice of my body was being replaced with new, fresh air, allowing joy back into my life. I could slowly feel the embers of my inner fire glowing hotter every day.

But now that I'd been on the road alone for three weeks, longing started to creep in. As much as I had an unstoppable desire to get away from everything, to be alone for a while, I wasn't expecting I'd miss my husband so much. By the end of the trip, if I made it, my whole body would be one expansive longing for Jim. Imagining the touch of his lips at the exact spot between my shoulder blades and the nape of my neck sent a shiver up my spine. That same spot, which was usually the source of the greatest pleasure, was burning with pain as I climbed endless miles. I had to keep going, so I could close the gap of time, before I could finally lie down next to the love of my life, feeling his arms wrapped tightly around my thinning body and his lips pressing against my back.

—FIFTEEN—
We See What We Want to See

Show me the way to go home.
I'm tired and I want to go to bed.
—sung by Johnny Diamond,
lyrics by Irving King

My skin prickled with fear and the anticipation of crossing into Mexico. It was Sunday, October 21, my twenty-fourth day on the road, and I was right where I thought I'd be, when I thought I'd be. I looked forward to riding in the desert, but I had my concerns. It is always the fear of the unknown that causes us discomfort. Because of this fear, we often don't venture out, and consequently, we are robbed of new and beautiful experiences that give our lives meaning. I knew I would have to be alert and smart. I hoped my Garmin cooperated and the maps would show me the way I was supposed to go. The Sierra Divide maps provided good practice, and Garmin tech support got me through the hurdles. I thought I was ready.

I left Calimesa at the foot of the San Bernardino mountain range, and sang the opening lyrics to myself from the famous Willie Nelson song "On the Road Again."

I didn't remember all the words, but now the melody stuck in my head, playing on the loop. Okay, Mr. Nelson—let's get on the road again. I navigated my way out of Calimesa and followed Cherry Lane to Beaumont. Would I have liked to ride through the wilderness this land had once been a long time ago? Sure. But this was now, and it was just a part of my journey. I was learning about places I'd never been. I left town as the wind started to pick up. I was preoccupied looking at the maps on my iPhone and my Garmin to make sure I stayed on track. I looked up, and a mountain rose before me, the road zigzagging back and forth into infinity and beyond.

Seriously!

Wasn't I done with big climbs and crossing mountain ranges? I put on my brave hat and started climbing. The wind whipped me and slapped me around like a wet towel. Several times it threw me off The Beast and forced me to walk. I wanted to scream!

I did. Loudly. Shrieking several times to release my frustration.

When I coached skiing, I always told the kids to relax. "Don't grip your poles so tight! Relax your shoulders. Close your eyes, breathe, and let the mountain guide you. Be light on your feet, feel the skis under you connected to your body. Calm down and control your emotions." I would teach young athletes how to visualize their runs at the start, and we would go through a series of relaxation exercises. Irony of ironies. Now I was telling myself those same things. Relaxing and softening the tight grip of my handlebars worked to some extent, but The Beast and I were like a bull in the ring attacking the wind ferociously. There was no shoulder, and some cars and trucks didn't really give me much space. I also got fewer of the honks and waves and thumbs-ups that usually gave me extra and much-needed motivation. It just seemed like people were driving faster and were in a bigger hurry to get to wherever they were going.

I was sitting by the side of the road, resting, eating trail mix, and drinking water when a truck passed. A big photo of a grinning

George Clooney whizzed by. It was a delivery truck for his tequila company.

"Come back, George! Come baaaaaaack!" I yelled after the truck and gave myself a good laugh. As I dreamed about Clooney, I decided my husband was much better looking. He is tall, broad-shouldered, and strong, with a lean muscular body and olive skin. I love running my hands through his thick salt-and-pepper hair. His eyes, the color of glacial lake melting on the sunny spring day, have just the right mix of shyness and authority, which take my breath away. Years ago, when I was just getting to know him, I ran into him and his daughter in the grocery store. I was standing in the line a few people back while they were already checking out. He looked back at me and held my gaze, a nasty habit of his that made my knees wobble. No doubt I had fallen for Jim's looks the minute I'd laid eyes on him. It's his honesty, loyalty, and unrelenting character that I love most about him, but his looks don't hurt.

The day after I received my cancer diagnosis, we went to have a meeting with my surgeon. It was our first time walking together into the cancer center. The heavy sliding door creaked open, and we entered holding hands, both stunned. Just months before, we had visited our nephew there, contemplating the unfairness of cancer affecting someone so young and innocent. The nurse showed us to the room, and the door shut behind. We waited for the doctor to arrive in uncomfortable silence. She entered with an easy and confident smile. Jim sat quietly, looking at his feet while I discussed my options with the surgeon. I almost forgot he was there, and for a moment, I thought he wasn't listening to the conversation. After she took me through the steps she asked, "How do you feel about doing the reconstructive surgery, Alenka? You will have a chance to rebuild your breasts just the way you want them to be. There are different options, but we won't know until we remove the tumor whether you need chemo, radiation, or both. That will determine the timing of reconstruction."

I was so overwhelmed by everything that I didn't know what to say. I wasn't ready for any of that. I hadn't done any research yet. I looked over at Jim.

"What do you think about all this?"

He didn't hesitate. He said my breasts were the least important thing to him: that all he wanted was for the doctor to keep me alive and well.

At that moment, it was all that I needed to hear from him. I knew he loved me for who I was, not the way I looked, and that was his way of saying it.

On my ride, alone in the tent at night, I missed placing my head on Jim's strong bare chest, inhaling his masculine scent, and having his arms wrapped around me.

My legs and back started cramping badly as I climbed, whipped mercilessly by wind. I pulled over and washed down an electrolyte pill. It was covered in pocket fuzzies, but I was glad to find it.

I was amazed at how adaptable my body was, despite the recent surgeries. I swore I could feel myself healing. Somehow, I'd made it through one day, then another and another. I was slowly rediscovering myself, slowly rekindling the embers of a dormant fire. If I just kept moving, I would eventually arrive, perhaps not where I'd planned, but I would always arrive somewhere.

As I continued my climb, I thought back to when my son was eleven years old. I had loaded a double kayak with food and camping gear and we'd taken off from the beach below our cabin to circumnavigate Lake Tahoe. I wanted to show him that adventure was possible in our backyard. Oh, he complained all right.

"Paddle!" I'd call out to him as we were zigzagging all over the place, going in circles. "We have to work together, or we'll never get anywhere."

He complained that he was too tired. By then, I was doing all the paddling. We finally synchronized our strokes and got better and better keeping an almost straight line, moving along, and making visible progress. We'd pull over and camp wherever we had a chance in little coves with no one around us. He loved gathering wood to build a small campfire under a starry sky and roasting hot dogs on a stick. On the last day, we had to cross a section of the lake that at first looked impossibly far. But slowly, trees on the other side of the lake gained shape. When we landed on the beach several hours later, it was amazing to see the joy, pride, and feeling of an accomplishment in my son's young eyes. We didn't land anywhere near where we thought we would, but we had the best camp spot nestled between the giant granite boulders on the east shore of the lake. We set up our tent, built sand forts, read books, fished without luck, and made a cozy home on our last day of the trip.

Just when I was feeling at my lowest, my body aching, I came upon a sign for a Zen center. It looked like a beautiful and peaceful place to stop, with sweeping vistas. I took time to regroup and sit and breathe for a while under the sign on the side of the road. I realized that if I slowed down for just a bit, I could see more clearly again. There was a reason for everything at the right time, at the right place.

I thought of my father's wise words from my childhood again.

"Stop and turn downhill," he used to advise me. "Look how far you've come, not how far you still have to go. See how much you've accomplished already and be proud of yourself!"

That's what I was doing. I was sitting down on the side of the road and looking back into the valley, and I felt proud of how far I'd come. My father's spirit was with me, and he would guide me over this last part of the climb for the day. I felt good.

That day I climbed thirty-four miles, 4,819.6 feet into ferocious winds, and spent eight hours, fourteen minutes, and thirteen seconds in the saddle. But I could not calculate the distance I'd traveled inside myself. It was immeasurable. With that sense of accomplishment propelling me, I reached Stone Creek campground in San Jacinto State Park at dusk. The hosts, Larry and Rita, were so helpful. They came to my campsite and started a fire for me. They also shined the headlights from their golf cart so I could quickly set up my tent. I boiled water, and the Top Ramen tasted delicious, mainly because I was so tired and cold. I sat by the fire for a while, watching stars and the moon which was waxing gibbous, just past the half-moon phase.

The winds were forecast to pick up even more during the night. I made sure the fire was completely out before I crawled into my tent and hoped I would stay reasonably warm and get some sleep. I had been celebrating being warm and done with big climbs a bit prematurely. I put away my mind's champagne bottles.

In the morning, I started a fire with pine needles and branches and made hot cocoa, oatmeal, and two quesadillas. I was tired and still hungry. I sat by the fire wrapped in my quilt, rested and wrote. I needed to sit the winds out.

Beautiful manzanita bushes flanked my campsite, and cedars surrounded me. They were much straighter and taller than the ones at home, which are all gnarled and twisted and low to the ground. I loved their twisting red branches adorned by contrasting bright green needles that hung like emerald jewels. I saw my life reflected in the trees. When a tree has the opportunity and room to grow, its branches straighten out and reach for the sky. I closed my eyes and listened to the wind above the crowns of the magnificent trees. It felt as if they were speaking directly to me. Birds sang morning prayers, and the Steller's jays squawked. I was in no hurry. I would pack slowly and head toward Idyllwild to see what was there. I stopped to say goodbye to campground hostess Rita. We talked about our kids, who were the same age, and then she reached for the pen and wrote her phone number on a piece of paper she tore out of her ledger book. She said she would worry about me and offered to come get me if anything went wrong. I thanked her and rode off.

Idyllwild is a lovely mountain town. In July 2018, the fast-moving Cranston fire burned thousands of acres and came incredibly close to taking out the town. An arson suspect was arrested shortly afterward.

I stopped at the Village Market to resupply; then, taking advantage of a signal, I chatted with Jim. I loved hearing his voice. I decided I would finally really have a rest day and only ride eight and a half more miles to the campground at Lake Hemet. It was still windy, so I was happy about the choice. The road went down and down and down, and I sang a happy tune to myself and enjoyed the warm wind on my face. I rode through the burn area, and it was scary to see how close to town the fire had come.

What is wrong with people? I thought out loud as I rode past charred trees.

I saw the lake not so far away and pulled over at a farm stand. My kind of a place. Back at Idyllwild market, I'd bought a pack of ravioli, and there at the farm stand I chose a couple of tomatoes and some basil. I looked forward to just sitting by the lake in the warm sun and could already picture myself with a beer and a yummy dinner.

At the farm stand, I started chatting with a guy and asked him if there was a store at Lake Hemet.

"You mean you are heading up that way?" He pointed at the road winding steeply back up the hill.

"What do you mean up that way? I just came from up there!"

"Well, you missed Lake Hemet!"

"How the hell could I have missed it?" I asked, bewildered.

Turns out, the lake I'd been looking at was not Lake Hemet, but Mystic Lake. I replayed the trip in my mind. Before I started my descent, I had stopped at the gas station at Mountain Center to get seventeen cents worth of fuel for my stove. In hindsight, I now recalled the road went to the left and up the hill. I had continued straight and down the mountain, without double-checking my maps. Because there was a lake at the bottom of my road, I'd assumed it must be Lake Hemet. I guess we see what we want to see.

The idea of riding back up the steep hill for eight miles made me nauseated.

I started hitchhiking. Was this foolish? Maybe. But I'm optimistic and hopeful by nature. And I had met with nothing but kindness on this trip so far. Besides, it was Friday. Lots of people were heading to the mountains. I was hoping someone with a pickup would have mercy. Several people waved, and I recognized the gesture. Oh, we'd love to, but we have no room! Sorry! They smiled and shrugged. I didn't blame them. They saw The Beast and me, and they thought, *Yeah right! No way we have room for that bike*!

I stood by the road with my hand and thumb extended, as campers and pickup trucks kept speeding by. I remembered then what Rita from the campground said: "Now if you need anything, anything at all," and I was so tempted to call her. She would have come too. She was that kind of person. But I couldn't have someone drive all the way down and all the way back up the mountain because I'd made a dumb mistake.

Just then, a blue pickup pulled in from the Idyllwild direction and stopped. I recognized it as one of the vehicles that had driven past me. The driver, Carlos, had turned around to come back for me. Carlos lived in Idyllwild, and after I explained to him that I had taken a wrong turn, he said, yes, of course, he could give me a ride back up the hill. He was a disabled vet with tattoos covering his arms, a leather vest with emblems, and an American flag bandanna—the proper outfit for a biker dude. The guy from the fruit stand helped us load my heavy bike into the back of Carlos's pickup. We had to rearrange his collection of a chainsaw, gas tanks, and a bunch of other tools to make room. The two seemed to know each other, which made me feel a tad safer.

On the way up the hill, Carlos did most of the talking. Back in 2004, he told me, he had walked the Appalachian Trail to raise money for his aunt, who had breast cancer. She was his favorite aunt, and she died during treatment. Recently, he said, he had crashed his Harley and was lucky to be alive. He'd just had an accident with his new truck. He was recently divorced. I listened to him and was so bloody grateful I was getting a ride back to where I was supposed to go. Just before he dropped me off, he told me he also volunteered at the children's hospital for kids with cancer.

That broke me wide open, and I teared up. After listening to his heartbreaking and compassionate stories, I confessed, "Carlos, the reason I am doing the ride is that I just went through breast cancer treatments myself. I am looking to rekindle my life and find faith in myself and the world around me." He looked at me in shock. "You are a good guy, Carlos! I am really sorry about your aunt."

Carlos wanted to say something, but he just sat there choking up.

"You made my day, not just because you gave me a ride," I told him before I gave him a hug goodbye. I didn't take pictures with him. I knew he'd stay in my memory just the way he was, a big burly guy with tattoos that rose from his chest, where the kindest heart resides. I will always remember the guy who turned around because he wanted to help a stranger in need.

I realized this was exactly what I had gone out to find. Something real that would show me that, yes, life can be good when you meet kind people.

—SIXTEEN—
Leaving It All Behind

I try to treat whoever I meet as an old friend. This gives me
a genuine feeling of happiness. It is the practice of compassion.
—His Holiness, the Dalai Lama

On my twenty-third day, I left Lake Hemet campground, which had cost me an outrageous fifty-four dollars. Carlos had dropped me off at the campground entrance and I ate dinner by the fire, trying to keep warm. The embers flying in the wind burned tiny holes in the Thermarest I was sitting on. Realizing how dangerous that was, I quickly smothered the fire with water. Several times during the night, I awoke on the hard ground and had to reinflate it. In the morning, I took time to patch the holes before starting off. I'd have to be careful in the desert with the thorns as well. As incredible as this new, lightweight equipment was, it was also very delicate. My tent was also whisper-light, and it flew out of my hands when I was setting it up in strong wind. Once I started camping in Baja, it was easy to imagine it getting wrapped around a *cardon* cactus.

I kept thinking about my ride with Carlos. Listening to him talking about his motorcycle crash brought back memories. I took off riding on Pines to Palms Highway 74, past Mount Thomas and beyond, thinking about the crash that had almost claimed the life of my eldest daughter, Mateja. That day—and the months that followed—were the most painful of my life. It's been six years since the accident. I remember it as if it were today.

I had been sitting in the garden with Tilen and two of our friends. Mateja had taken Jim's perfectly restored 1957 Chevy truck to the weekly farmers' market, part of the display we used to sell Tahoe Teas. We expected her back any moment for lunch and hilarious stories about who and what she had seen at the market. Instead, I received a text from my daughter Jana. She and her sister had been planning to drive to Reno to see a movie. It wasn't like Mateja not to respond. Before I could text her back, my phone rang. Jana said the customers coming into the resort where she worked had begun talking about a terrible accident on Highway 89 and that the road was closed. There was panic in her voice. I tried to calm her down, but I had that twisted feeling in my gut, the immediate mother's intuition that something was terribly wrong.

Our friends had left. To distract myself, I decided to cut Tilen's hair. We were out on the deck when the phone rang again. As soon as it did, I knew what was coming. There was just something about that ring. When I saw it was Jim calling, my fears were confirmed. Jim never calls me during the day while he is working. I didn't want to hear what he had to say, but he kept talking.

"The truck," he said, his voice thick with emotion, "The truck was in the accident!"

I had an out-of-body experience. Time froze. As it did, I watched myself standing on the deck, holding the phone and the scissors. I was frantic.

"No, no, not my baby," I heard myself say. "Please, not her!"

Jim promised to call back as soon as he had more information.

The phone rang again. It was my toll-free business number. Just to distract myself, I answered. The man on the other side of the line was in clear distress, telling me he just left the scene of the accident.

"It's horrible. Really bad," he kept repeating.

I couldn't stand to keep listening. I told him I had to go and hung up the phone. Just then, Jim called back.

Everything around me stopped moving.

"They flew her to the hospital in Reno," he said. "Here's the number for you to call. I'll pick you up in town."

Tahoe is a small community where everyone knows one another. Several firefighters and paramedics who had gone to the scene of the accident recognized our truck. Somehow, the news reached Jim at his job site in Alpine Meadows, right above the scene of the crash. Earlier, he had seen the local Life Flight helicopter circle above him. He did not know Mateja was on that flight.

Just a week before the accident, Jim had installed a three-point seatbelt on the truck. It undoubtedly saved Mateja's life. She had been driving home when a van in the opposing lane overshot the turn and plowed head-on into the truck. The van was full of kids who'd been attending summer wrestling camp, with a twenty-one-year-old boy driving. The passengers had been arguing about what to play on the radio station, and the young driver was distracted. The force of the impact pushed the Chevy's engine block into the cabin, leaving no more than ten inches for Mateja, who somehow slithered into the tiny gap under the dashboard.

There was incredible confusion at the scene. At first, all attention was on the boys in the van. Luckily, they all walked away with just minor scrapes and bruises, which was a miracle. The man first on the scene of the accident (who had called on my business number) told me later that he had climbed through the back window into the cab of the pickup and lifted Mateja's head from a pool of blood. She took a breath, and at that moment, came back to life. Otherwise, she would have drowned in her own blood.

After Jim gave me the number to the hospital, it took several deep breaths to calm myself enough to make the call. My only comforting thought was that Mateja was still alive. I told myself that they were flying her to the hospital. She would be okay.

The nurse on the phone confirmed that Mateja had arrived. She said her injuries included a broken femur and a broken arm.

We can deal with that, I thought, but my mind kept switching back to the distressed call from the man who was at the scene: "It's bad. It's terrible! I am so sorry!"

Was there something the nurse wasn't telling me?

I went out into the yard and screamed. I was afraid if I stopped talking, everything else would stop. I wanted to summon the higher powers to take over.

"Don't you dare take her!" I shouted to the heavens. "Take over! Now is the time if you are there! I need you!"

It was an act of pure desperation. For the first time in my life, I needed God to exist. It was a hot August day, but I was suddenly cloaked in a veil of cold air.

"Go away!" I screamed.

I quickly went into survival mode, packing things up for what I already knew would be a long stay in the hospital.

After instructing Tilen to pack his things, I went to take a shower and packed bags for Jim and Jana as well. When I think about it now, I think I was subconsciously trying to delay the departure to deal with the inevitable.

A friend brought Jana from her job. We met Jim at the Save Mart parking lot, and he drove us to Reno. I was calm on the outside as I told them, "It's just a broken arm and femur. She'll be okay." Yet, on the inside, I could hardly breathe. Time was twisted like a gnarly tree on a mountaintop blasted by the winds. It stretched in all directions, and I was spinning in it. I felt as if I were levitating in my seat. I talked to Mateja and told her to hang in there, that we were on our way.

At the hospital, they took us immediately to see her. Seeing my child on the gurney wearing an oxygen mask and covered in tubes, her head and face swollen and barely recognizable, sucked the life out of me.

"Hi, Mom," I could recognize her look. Her eyes were so big, so blue! She was scared and confused, but by then, the pain meds had begun to work, and she was very dazed. The fact that she recognized me instantly gave me hope. I tried to reassure her but was probably just reassuring myself and everyone else. I'm still not sure. My body stood there, my mouth was talking to the doctors and nurses, but I, again, seemed to be levitating and watching the scene from above.

This is not happening to us. I want to lie down and take your place. I want to take your pain, your suffering, your fear.

Every parent watching their child going through trauma knows this feeling.

The first report from the doctor was that she had a broken femur, broken arm and clavicle, broken facial bones, broken ribs, punctured lungs, and—the scariest of it all—bleeding on the brain. The doctor warned that, if swelling increased, they would have to surgically remove part of her skull to alleviate the pressure. My blood curdled at the thought.

"The CAT scan will show more later," the doctor told us, "but she has to go into surgery for the broken femur immediately." As she was wheeled away from me, we got swept into the rhythm of life within hospital walls, not knowing where the journey would take us or how long it would last.

Mateja's stepmother, Kristen, was a nurse. She had been working as head nurse in another hospital near the crash that day. A dispatch call came in about the accident, followed by a highway patrol officer who arrived just ahead of the boys in the van. The officer told Kristen that the other crash victim was being flown to Reno with multiple injuries and severe head trauma. He showed Kristen Mateja's driver's license, not realizing she was her stepmom. Kristen called Tom, my ex-husband, Mateja's dad, who was driving home from Salt Lake City. I'm sure the rest of the trip was agony for him.

The CHP officer arrived just as Mateja was wheeled into ICU from her first of many surgeries. "I'd like to talk with you," he said in a low voice.

I sure as hell was not ready to talk to anyone in a uniform at that moment. The last thing I wanted to hear was that the accident was Mateja's fault. He must have read that on my face because he insisted again, saying it would just take a minute. I agreed and slid onto the cold, shiny hospital floor, smelling of disinfectant. I leaned my back against the wall and closed my swollen eyes.

"I think you'll want to know it was not Mateja's fault," he told me. "It might not be important to you right now, but it will matter later."

I thanked him. But he still had more to say.

"I'm glad to see your daughter is still alive. I'm sorry she was in such a terrible accident, but I think she'll pull through."

Mateja's first surgery lasted several hours. Before they wheeled her into the operating room, a young handsome orthopedic surgeon assured me that he would be cautious about saving the tattoo on her right hip. It says *Credendo Vides* which means "by believing, one sees." The saying is from Mateja's favorite book, *Voyage of the Basset*, which I read to her when she was a little girl. It's a richly illustrated book about the journey of a young girl on the good ship *Bassett* as it sails into a mystical world, in which magical kingdoms emerge from the sea of dreams.

I told him I didn't care at all about the tattoo. I just wanted her to be well. He shook his head.

"Trust me. She will care."

I hoped that was a good sign. You can only care about a tattoo if you are alive, right?

Watching my child being wheeled into surgery was like ripping my heart out. The daughter of the flight nurse who had treated Mateja was on the ski team I coached. He recognized Mateja immediately, and after his shift, he came to the ICU to check on us. He seemed almost as happy as I was that she was still alive.

"She went into a fight-or-flight response. As small as she is, we could hardly hold her down," he told me. "She's a fighter. She'll make it."

I found it impossible to sleep for the next week. I sat in the chair next to Mateja night and day. One night, a young male nurse came to change her dressing around the tube they had inserted into her collapsed lung. Mateja looked like she was sleeping and not aware of what was going on. As he peeled off the surgical tape on her chest, she bolted upright.

"You motherfucker! That hurts!" she screamed through the oxygen mask.

The nurse jumped back, knocking over a cart, scattering everything on the floor. He looked at me in shock. It was the first time I'd smiled in days.

"That's my girl," I told him. "She's small, but she's feisty. Don't mess with her."

I knew right then that she would survive. It would take time to make her whole again, but she would come back to us. The nurse and I couldn't help but laugh. It was the laughter of relief and surrender at the same time.

In that moment of crisis, we all came together. Mateja's stepmom was invaluable. We were all in a state of shock, especially during the first days in the ICU when Mateja was still in critical condition. Kristen guided us through the process. She instructed us what to look for and how to communicate with the doctors and nurses. Different doctors and nurses rotated through her room day and night. It was challenging to keep track, but we caught many things that nurses might have missed.

One of the first things Mateja asked when she became aware of her situation many days later was, "What happened to my tattoo?" I was happy to tell her that the good doctor did a fantastic job saving it. She smiled and sank back into her fantasy world while monitors beeped and blue lights glared. I continued to exist in my half-waking state. I was turning into a zombie, but I couldn't leave her side.

I fed Mateja clear broth spoon by spoon, just like when she was my little baby.

Afterward, she closed her eyes to rest. I just sat there with the spoon in my hand, staring at her swollen face, her bandaged head, and the tubes attached to every part of her body. I was breathing in the rhythm of the beeping monitors that connected me with my daughter as if we were still connected by the umbilical cord.

In time, a therapist came to test Mateja's cognitive, fine motor skills, and memory. She asked Mateja to write down the name of her favorite author. The letters, which were barely legible, were scattered across the page from the bottom left toward the upper right corner of the page. The therapist asked me to write my own answers, so we could compare. I wrote down "Jonathan Franzen," one of our favorite writers. I was hoping she would do the same. On the morning of her accident, I had finished reading "My Father's Brain," from Franzen's book of essays, *How to Be Alone*, which Mateja had gifted me. We had talked about that essay over breakfast, just before she drove off to the farmers' market. When the therapist told me Mateja had written his name, I wanted to kiss Franzen on the lips.

Time became a blur of a different kind, now a span of blinking lights and beeping alarms. But at least in this facility I had my own plastic futon where I could sleep next to her.

One night, I must have drifted off to sleep when I heard the beeping of her bed signal, which meant she was planning to escape out of bed. I bolted awake in time to see her hunting for her clothes.

"Okay, Mom, time to get dressed," she told me. "Time to go to church."

It took me a few seconds to orient myself. It took a few more to remember we don't go to church. But she was insistent. We were on our way to ten o'clock mass. Whose or where, I had no idea. We almost never went to church, except on Easter or Christmas or when we were back in the Old Country.

I looked at my watch and saw that it was one fifteen. I adjusted Mateja's oxygen tubes and gently massaged her feet. Eventually, she fell back to sleep, but I was wide awake. I stood by her side for a long time, watching her face glowing in a blue night-light.

Just when I was about to return to my hard futon, a morning nurse arrived and woke Mateja to take her vitals. I've never understood why they can't just let a patient sleep, especially one with brain injuries.

The nurse was still checking Mateja's blood pressure when she suddenly remembered where we were supposed to be headed.

"Mom, get the clothes ready," she insisted. "We have to go to church at ten. I told you. They really want me to thank them."

"Who are *they*, Mateja? Did you have a dream?"

No, insisted Mateja. Vampires might be imaginary, but these guys (whoever they may have been) were real.

"I want my nice clothes," she demanded. "I want to look pretty. Please get me my makeup; I need to cover up my raccoon eyes."

It was so hard to see her like that. Was she somehow suspended between reality and her dream world, or was it the in-between world? Did they really come to see her? The ones who saved her? Had she crossed over, and then when her head was lifted out of the pool of blood, was she able to take a breath and return?

I was so shaken by what she was saying that a flood of tears streamed down my cheeks, but there was no sound coming out of me. Just hot, wet tears, flowing as if they belonged to someone else. It was me now, thanking the ones who had brought my baby back to me.

The doctor in charge at Reno Renown Hospital was ready to release her after two terrifying and exhausting weeks in ICU. We insisted she needed further medical attention, so we had her transferred to UC Davis facility in Sacramento with the help of our friends Tim and Suzanne. Mateja's multiple injuries were so severe that some went undetected until we requested additional MRIs and CAT scans. I would arrive at five each morning and catch doctors on their first rotation. It was the only time one was able to see and talk with the doctors before they went into surgery for the rest of the day. I would then walk back to my friends Tim's and Suzan's house and cook food to take to Mateja for lunch and dinner. She hated hospital food. Nurturing my child by cooking her favorite meals often seemed the only way I could be helpful.

Mateja required multiple surgeries and months in rehab facilities. She was in a wheelchair for months after that. From the orthopedic department, she was transferred to a rehab department to deal with her brain injuries. I'd sit in the background, taking notes during her therapy sessions. Her severe head trauma had sheared connections between axons and neurons in her brain. Scientists have learned a lot about the brain's capacity to regenerate, but the recovery level was still a great unknown. In Mateja's case, her handwriting and her speech were slowly improving. Between naps, we'd play cards and word games, like Scrabble and Bananagrams. Soon she started winning. When she rested, I'd read her favorite books to her. We laughed like two crazy girls, and we'd both fall asleep exhausted. Those were our days.

The physical therapy nurses taught me how to slide her into the wheelchair from bed and load her into and out of the car. With both legs and an arm in casts, she was only able to wrap one arm around my neck to help me lift her. We were able to go on our first outing weeks later to sit by the pool at our friends' house. Their son Jenner, a few months younger than Tilen, had started playing rugby in high school and worked out all the time. He was buff. When we arrived at their house, he picked Mateja out of the car and just carried her like a doll to their backyard. It was Mateja's first time outside in fresh air under the bright sun. I enjoyed just sitting there, watching the kids joke with each other and play cards. It was so good to hear their laughter again. Life felt almost normal for an hour.

We were learning to navigate through life in a wheelchair. The next outing was to the movies. Mateja was excited at first to be able to go out, but that quickly changed when we entered the mall full of people. "Why is everyone staring at me?" she asked.

I could tell she was suffering.

"I hate it. I hate being in a wheelchair."

She was angry. And it broke my heart to watch my daughter, who had lived such an independent life, feeling stuck and helpless, dependent on me and everyone else around her. The whole purpose in raising your kids is to prepare them to live their own lives. Mateja had already traveled all over the world, studied in Europe, and was on her way to earning her master's degree from Mills College in English and comparative literature.

There were times she hated me as well and was often angry when I tried to help her get dressed. She hated me when I'd have to remind her friends who were visiting that it was time for them to leave so she could rest, which was essential for her brain recovery. She had been a fiercely independent and stubborn child. When she turned three, she just refused to get dressed in the mornings, especially when we were hurrying out the door. It would take two people to pin her down and get her dressed, while she was screaming and kicking. This very challenging trait, which made her such a difficult toddler, a stubborn child, and later a rebellious teenager, was most beneficial when she was fighting her way back after the accident. Often a very fine line separates us from crossing into eternal life. For reasons unknown, some make a U-turn and return to life on Earth.

Many months after the crash, Mateja took her first unassisted steps on the sandy beaches in Baja, just below our palapa. Baja is our healing place. After a year of hard work and pure determination, she returned to Mills College and graduated with honors. It is our job as parents to care for and teach our children. In that crucial period, though, I drew strength and learned from how my own children handled the trauma. There was no time for despair. We all just had to put one foot in front of another, and it brought us closer.

Years later, on my epic ride from Tahoe to Mexico, I was finally able to process the events. It was as if the roles were reversed. Mateja has been my main link to family and friends on this trip. Often, she and I would chat on the phone as I was lying in the tent exhausted. She would comfort me and encourage me to endure. I sent her updates as often as I could, so she could post them to my blog. This way my friends and my family were able to follow my progress and my experiences.

Many thoughts ran through my mind when I was riding. I often had to pull to the side of the road to write notes on my phone. I'd stand there, bracing the bike between my legs, afraid to take time to get off my bike. If I didn't write down what I was thinking right then and there, my thoughts evaporated. I wrote when I stopped for lunch and when I lay in bed. I was able to write because I was moving, seeing, feeling everything around me and everything within me. Riding along a lonely road where I didn't have to pay attention to traffic or anything else allowed my thoughts and memories to take over. I remembered. I processed. I shed pain from the past. Moving farther down the road was my salvation.

—SEVENTEEN—
The Kindness of Strangers

You can always, always give something,
even if it is only kindness.
—Anne Frank

It was day twenty-five of my trip. I was on The Beast by nine in the morning, hoping to reach the Southern California town of Campo, just along the Mexican border.

I still had so many miles to cover. I stopped by a gas station and heated a frozen breakfast burrito in a microwave. I sipped hot coffee while I waited and chatted with the clerk. I wished I could stay and get to know her better.

Originally from New Jersey, Marion had moved West in the '70s. Her eyes, the color of lapis reflecting the deep California sky, shone brightly. She was one of those people with whom you forge an instant connection and wish you could sit and talk forever. She asked me if I was afraid of going into Mexico by myself. I told her I knew I should have been after all the warnings I'd received, but that they just didn't square with my experience.

"The news is full of sensational stories, drug cartels, gangs, and murders," I said. "But all the Mexican people I have encountered are honest, kind, and helpful. So, no, I am not going to allow myself to be worried."

She nodded her head. "That's exactly how I feel."

"We are all like animals," I philosophized further. "If we are fearful, distrustful, judgmental, or hateful, other people pick that up just like an animal would. They will act accordingly." I smiled and added, "I'm hoping I'm proved right on this journey."

We both agreed that maybe we were naive, but that if you see the good in the person in front of you, if you don't judge by their appearance, they will find good in you in return, no matter where you are in the world.

"I think you're right," Marion said, her blue eyes shining even brighter, "we are all just human animals."

I wanted to keep talking. But I had to keep moving. Marion and I hugged, and I rode off.

Again, I was powered up hills by the love of the people I met. The Beast and I made a beautiful long climb toward the town of Julian. By the time I reached the outskirts, I'd already climbed 1,800 feet and peddled twenty miles. I passed many signs that claimed BEST APPLE PIE or GRANDMA'S PIE. I was obviously in apple country and during peak apple picking season. I pulled over at a barn-like complex that had a bunch of vendors. There was everything from antique shops to a hard cider bar and a taco restaurant, which was what I'd stopped for. I was ready for some food.

The taco restaurant was still closed, so I ventured into a "Honey Fermented" drink bar run by Jessie and his wife. Jessie was a big guy adorned with tattoos, and he jumped into his sales pitch as soon as I sat down at the counter: "Would you like to taste a flight of mead? We offer delicious aged-fermented honey wine ranging from eight to fifteen percent alcohol. You can mix any flavors we offer." He finally took a breath.

"I'm on my way to the border and farther down the Baja Peninsula," I said, to explain my reason for not being able to try more than one sample. "I'm trying to make it to Campo tonight!"

He couldn't quite believe it.

"I have a funny story for you!" he said excitedly. "A couple of years back, I was going to get back in shape." He put both hands on his belly and jiggled it, laughing. "I decided to ride my bike to work from my house in town three miles up the hill. Well, this is fun, I say to myself riding down the hill. But then, on my way home, it's all uphill. I got halfway home and called my wife to come get me with the truck!" He looked over at his wife. "Right, honey?"

We all laughed. When I went back out to the taco restaurant, the line was twenty people deep. Where did all these people come from? I joined the line, as it was the only food place in the complex. It looked and smelled delicious, so I waited. I was starving. I finally reached the counter and ordered a taco plate. A kid at the register said, "No need to pay."

"Pardon me?"

He said again, "Your lunch has already been paid for by Jessie."

I was stunned by the unexpected gesture. I sat at the counter, and once again, quiet tears of gratitude rolled down my cheeks. I knew it looked weird with all the people around me, but I couldn't help it. Even if I were to quit the trip right then and there, I would have accomplished the most important part of my journey. My faith in humanity had been restored.

On my way out, I walked by Jessie's place and waved goodbye to him. He was busy with customers, so I just mouthed my words from the door in his direction, *Thank you!* He toasted a glass in my direction and mouthed back, *Good luck!*

I was excited and nervous to be approaching the border. What if all the people who had warned me were right? What if I was just stupid and naive? Maybe I should wait and ride across the border with someone, like they were advising cyclists to do?

After forty-two miles and 4,537 feet of climbing, I happily reached Laguna Mountain Lodge. I decided to stay at the lodge so I could log onto Wi-Fi to review my border crossing notes one last time. I checked the Baja Divide website: the crossing itself looked straightforward, but I was concerned. I read the posted warning several times:

"Due to a number of incidents in the previous two seasons of the Baja Divide in the Tecate area, riders were advised to remain on the main highway, MEX3, to the small community of San Francisco, which is 14.7 km or 9.1 miles from the US/MX border crossing. To the best of my knowledge," continued Nicholas Carman, who developed the Baja Divide route along with Lael Wilcox in the winter of 2015-2016, "at least four incidents have been reported in or near Tecate in those two years, mostly involving lone male assailants. All reports indicate money and valuables were the target of theft, and no physical assaults have been reported, although in several cases a gun has been reported to be involved and physical violence has been threatened."

I also read the news about two experienced male cyclists traveling around the world. Holger was from Germany, Krysztof from Poland. They were both reported missing by their families and later found brutally murdered. Their mutilated bodies were found not far apart from each other in the ditch on the side of the road. I regretted reading about all that. It made me very uneasy. Most of all, I really hoped Jim wouldn't come across those articles. I was afraid if he did, he would not allow me to continue with my ride across the border, and I was afraid I'd have to agree with him for all our sakes.

—EIGHTEEN—
The Moment of Truth

Love of one's country is a splendid thing.
But why should love stop at the border?
—Pablo Casals, Spanish musician

woke up at four thirty. It was still dark, but I knew I wouldn't be able to go back to sleep. I caught up on my writing, took a shower, and practiced some yoga to calm my nerves. When I sat on the towel, I noticed that my left quad was much larger than my right one. I'd been hoping that after all this hard riding, the muscles of my damaged right leg would start to kick in. It was just another reason for going on this ride. No physical therapy, meds, or time passing had helped so far. I took my earbuds cord to measure the circumference of my quad in a couple of places, and I came more than an inch short on my right side. My left side was compensating so much for the damage on my right that I was going to look as lopsided as a hunchback by the time I reached Southern Baja.

Monday, October 22, was my twenty-sixth straight day of riding. As The Beast and I departed the Cleveland National Forest, the road was quiet except for the chirping of thousands of birds. Golden oak trees lined the road. I was in a great mood, giddy with excitement to cross the border. I greeted every tree and every little bird that flew by me.

"Winter is coming!" I called out to the birdies. "Eat up, get fat, and fly south! I'll meet you down in Baja!"

I sang a Slovenian song from my favorite childhood movie, *Kekec*, in which a brave young boy merrily walks on a mountain path, singing:

"Kaj mi poje ptičica, ptičica sinička?
Dobra volja je najbolja, to si piši za uho,
Mile jere, kisle cmere z nami vštric ne pojdejo."

"What is the little bird singing to me? The little bird chickadee?
With good spirits is the way to go. This you always ought to know!
The crying and the weak, with us in step will never keep!"

The song has a happy, catchy tune, which I hummed and whistled, flying downhill. I was so happy that I was finally descending, that I waved at every passing car. People probably thought I was crazy, but I didn't care. I even waved at a black vehicle that had official red and blue lights flashing. Oops!

After less than an hour, I crossed Highway 8 and turned left onto the historic Highway 80. Passing the first border control, I greeted the two patrol guys, one tall and skinny, blond and sullen-looking; the other short, stout, and dark-haired with a Hispanic accent.

"How far to the border?"

"Five miles," they replied.

Five miles? That didn't make sense.

I asked again, "How far is the Tecate border crossing?"

"Oh, Tecate! That's about thirty miles."

It was clear they were accustomed to patrolling this area on foot, looking for people who illegally crossed the mountains in front of us. As I rode off, I subconsciously searched the hills, looking to see if I could spot anyone. How desperate must one be to risk their life crossing the border over such difficult terrain? How many desperate parents and their children have lost their lives?

I soon turned off Highway 80 toward Campo. The road was quiet and beautiful, granite boulders lining both sides of the narrow road. It was a good thing I hadn't made it to Campo the previous night. Apart from a railroad museum, a general store, and an old army barracks built during World War II to house prisoners of war, there was no suitable place to camp as far as I could see. It was practically a ghost town. Riding alongside the corrugated metal half wall, knowing that it was separating people, gave me a very strange and eerie feeling. The road was quiet but creepy. The only cars that passed me were a few border patrol cars. It was all so surreal. Borders separating us, guarding us, protecting us. From what? The walls and the borders in Europe were being erased. The walls that, in some cases, had separated people for centuries had come down. In the US, we were arguing about building higher, stronger walls so we could keep people out.

After forty-eight miles, I arrived at the border. I was able to reach Jana by phone to let her know and asked her to wish me luck. I told her I'd call everyone as soon as I found a place to spend the night in Tecate.

I walked my bike on the pedestrian side. The Mexican border guard directed me back to the office to get a tourist visa. I had to leave the bike outside, and that made me very uncomfortable. I tried to reassure myself: *I'm being stupid, thinking something might happen to The Beast. There are all these people around.* Nevertheless, I still locked my bike to the fence on the side of the building. I felt like a mother abandoning her baby. But then, that too struck me as absurd.

How many mothers and fathers have been separated from their children along this very border!

I walked into the office, and the official there was a chatty guy. I wanted to show off my Spanish, and he spoke back in perfect English. He said he'd love to visit Slovenia after hearing my descriptions of my beautiful homeland. "Do you have a sister back home I could marry?" He asked me. Oh, the charming Latin man!

Everyone warned me not to cross alone. But here I was. I put on my reading glasses to line up tiny numbers on my ultralight orange colored lock to unlock the bike. As I was pushing The Beast through heavy metal gates, I remembered how, as teenagers, we used to smuggle Levi's jeans in our ski bags, returning from ski training in Italy. We tried not to look guilty. We didn't want to declare what we'd bought, so we wouldn't have to pay an import tax. The guards somehow always let us pass.

A border guard on Mexico's side greeted me with a happy, "Welcome to Mexico" without ever taking his eyes off The Beast. I passed under a huge green, white, and red MEXICO sign, and that was it. I was on the other side, in a different country. And yet, I was still breathing the same air I had breathed on the other side of this so-called treacherous border.

I saddled The Beast and took a deep breath, trying not to think of reports of muggings and the murders I'd read about just this morning. I looked at the map on my phone and started riding toward the center square of Tecate. After so many days on backroads, the Technicolor scene was overwhelming: traffic, honking, music, color, aromas. Loud noise everywhere penetrated my skin, causing my whole body to vibrate from within. Souped-up cars with windows rolled down blasted music, I wondered if the person inside was deaf.

After two short blocks, I reached the central plaza of a typical bustling Mexican city. I immediately felt at home. I rode a couple of laps around the plaza. A modern Tecate brewing company building with its large tower and huge TECATE sign loomed above the scene. I wanted to see what else was around, rode some narrow streets lined by all kinds of odds-and-ends stores, bars and restaurants, and returned to the plaza where I had seen the Hotel Tecate earlier. I wanted to stay in the center, feel the vibe of the town. I was in freaking Mexico! Finally!

I found the entrance to the hotel, which was a bit tricky because of construction, and walking the bike over a two-by-eight plank took some balance. A couple of guys digging a trench below looked up at The Beast and me, and I just smiled and waved at them. They smiled back, waved, and returned to their digging. The hotel manager helped me carry the bike up the stairs. He kept shaking his head in amazement.

"Una bicicleta pesada! ¿Hasta donde vas?" (A heavy bike! Where are you going?)

"Montando en mi bicicleta a La Ventana, al sur de La Paz!" (I'm riding my bike to La Ventana, South of La Paz.)

"¿Sola?" (Alone?)

He was bewildered and concerned.

"Si, sola." (Yes, alone.)

I wondered if I was completely nuts to ride by myself. Even people here in Mexico think it's crazy. His elderly mother was sitting in the dimly lit office in a wheelchair, watching Spanish novellas on a small TV, a program equivalent to American soap operas. She looked up, and her toothless smile brightened. She waved at me as I passed by, pushing my bike. I grinned back, wanting to go over to give her a big hug. Walking along a narrow, dimly lit hallway, I reached my room, which was the last one on the right. I unlocked the door, and entered, awkwardly maneuvering The Beast ahead of me. My room was above a very busy street. I closed the window to shut out as much noise as the single glass pane could. Without taking off my tight, sweaty bike shoes and sweaty clothes, I lay prostrate on a lumpy, stiff bed that had a faint smell of cigarette smoke. A simple wooden cross above the bed was the only decoration in the room, which was painted the color of pink marshmallow. I immediately fell asleep.

When I awoke, I looked at my cell phone and realized I'd only slept for fifteen minutes. It felt as if I had been gone in dreamland for a very, very long time. I quickly sent a message to Jim, the kids, and my parents announcing my safe arrival, then showered. The stream was barely a trickle, so it took me a while to rinse out my hair. I washed it with multipurpose Castile camping soap. You can use it for washing the dishes or your dirty underwear. Afterward, my hair felt like dried yellow straw that even a cow wouldn't want to eat. I gave up trying to run my comb through it and instead put on a shirt I hadn't worn in a couple days, which made it that day's "clean" shirt. Next, I washed my bike liner shorts, socks, and the shirt I'd been sweating in for a few days and hung everything to dry over the bed frame.

After my chores were done, I chained my bike to the bed frame and locked the door behind me. I felt ridiculous taking these precautions. All the fears and anticipation of being in Mexico were so far unfounded. They began to fade away as I set out to explore the plaza.

Of course, I had to stay vigilant, just like in any city in the world. But the people I encountered here were just walking by, minding their own business. I was the one who looked odd and out of place. I was the one who received strange looks.

In truth, I stood out walking around in my bike shorts, flip-flops, and messy blond hair. I found a bank to get some pesos, then tucked into some headcheese tacos (what part of the cow's head remains a mystery). I lingered while a Mariachi band played and tipped them fifty pesos before heading out. Afterward, I walked around a bit, checking out barbershops, electronic stores with techno music blasting, dress shops with cream-colored quinceañera ball gowns displayed in the windows, and dulcerías with delicious pastries and sweets staring back at me.

In 1994, Daniel Reveles, an American writer born to Mexican parents and living in outskirts of Tecate, described Tecate as "a dusty little border town stippled with Easter-egg-colored houses where sovereign nations meet *panza*-to-*panza*. They are separated by four thin strands of rusty barbed wire. On Mondays, Señora Mendoza uses it for a clothesline. On a windy day I've seen her crawl through the wires and retrieve her underwear which has entered the United States illegally."

The Tecate of Reveles's stories seemed long gone. I crossed a much more heavily patrolled border. And in the place of those dusty, stippled streets were now blocks with a decidedly cosmopolitan feel. Just below my hotel was a fancy coffee shop bar called Paris. I treated myself to a delicious hot chocolate and cake. I couldn't resist. Just a pinch of guilt went through me, as I knew the cancer meant I shouldn't have sweets. But I was celebrating: a new country, new territory, new maps, a whole new adventure. I felt absolutely content.

The coffee shop was very urbane. People were dressed to the nines, and I sat there in my bike shorts and jacket, with hair looking like a haystack. I got some deserved funny looks. I didn't really care though, as I sat by myself, sipping hot chocolate and writing in my leather-bound notebook. I was distracted by people-watching and still amazed that I was in Mexico.

That night I had a very restful sleep. Just the fact that I'd made it that far felt like an accomplishment. I thought, after all the anticipation and nervousness, I was able to finally relax. My room was sparse; pink walls, a wooden cross above the bed that was stiff at best—but I was safe. I woke to the sound of church bells at quarter to eight, and was amazed I'd slept that long.

Packing up quickly, I headed to the same restaurant for a huevos rancheros breakfast, which came with chips, salsa, fresh avocado, and vegetable soup. All for six dollars, including coffee. The Mariachi band was still asleep somewhere—just like much of the city.

Ruta de Vino 3 took The Beast and me out of town toward Ensenada. As I began to peddle, an eighteen-year-old boy, who introduced himself as Diego Maximilian, joined me on his classic Schwinn bicycle. He was filled with all kinds of questions. At first, I was uneasy and kept checking to see whether there was anyone following us. Diego just rode alongside me, checking out my bike and pressing me for details only a fellow lover of adventure would want to know.

Practicing my Spanish, I learned from Diego that he was on his way home from selling burritos. His older brother made them, and every morning at four o'clock, Diego went to the bus station to sell them to the workers heading to the vineyards.

"I am a student, my last year of high school," he told me.

"What are your plans afterward?" I asked.

"My dad wants me to go to university, but my brother and I want to open a restaurant," he said enthusiastically.

"Go to university and study hard!" I told him. "Then you and your brother will have the best restaurant in town.

I promised to look him up once he opened his restaurant.

Before we parted ways, I oiled and cleaned his chain.

"You have a nice classic bike, Diego. Take care of it every day, and you'll have it for a long time."

I could tell he was proud of his wheels. For my part, I was glad to have made another new friend. He rode with me all the way to the outskirts of Tecate—about five miles—before we snapped photos, exchanged Facebook info, and parted ways.

After ten miles, I turned off the main road in the town of San Francisco, my last opportunity to resupply before entering the mountains. There would be no place to get water for at least sixty-three miles.

Hello world, hello, quiet dirt road, hello self and peace within me, I thought as I headed out again. *Hello, spirits of the ancient people of Kumeyaay, who roam free in these mountains. I hope you welcome me and protect me. I am here for you to show me the way. Help me find the new path to my inner self. Show me the remedies to heal my body and my soul. Cleanse my body of all these chemicals and let me be reborn.* A herd of beautiful, spirited horses ran alongside me for a while. I felt like a modern-day cowgirl, wishing to ride the black stallion among them.

I stopped in the shade of a giant ironwood tree after climbing a couple thousand feet on a beautiful dirt road. Closing my eyes, all I heard was the wind, a solitary bird, and a fly buzzing around my face. This was the Baja I had come to discover. This was the self I have come to unlock and set free.

The road climbed and wound through the rugged mountainside, then dropped to a meadow where tall pines grew. I passed sheep and cattle ranches as the shadows got longer, and my water supply dwindled. I should have stopped earlier and asked for some at a ranch I passed, but I'd chickened out. I was sure I'd pass another ranch soon. The rutted road rattled my brains and every bone in my battered body for a good part of the day.

I kept riding as the air finally cooled. It must have been close to six o'clock, judging by the sun that had long passed the horizon. The temperature was perfect, so I was able to cover more miles. I drank less water when the sun wasn't glaring down on me. I looked to my left, checking out a mass of granite boulders just as a giant orange full moon rose from behind the mountain, welcoming my arrival to the land of magic. I was soon bouncing mercilessly along a washboard road by the light of the full moon.

My son, Tilen, texted me: "Mom, are you still riding? Isn't it dark already?"

I texted back: "Yes, I am riding by the light of the moon, and an owl is keeping me company."

It warmed my heart to know Tilen was looking after me, but I also didn't want him to worry. I wished he were riding with me. It would have been nice to have his company at that moment. I missed my son, my best buddy. Since I coached his soccer, skiing, and mountain biking for so many years, we have had a very special bond. I knew he would have enjoyed this adventure. Riding alone in this remote area in Mexico, yet still close enough to the border where there were reports of muggings, my apprehensive imagination was trying to get the better of me. I started seeing funny shapes in the trees. I brushed against a branch I hadn't seen in the dark and thought someone was trying to grab me. A bird cackled and took off into the night. A chill entered my body, and I shivered all over.

After I had ridden for a couple more hours, the moon passed over and hid behind the mountain ridges, and now darkness pursued The Beast and me. The temperature dropped rapidly. It was that time of the night when I got anxious about where I'd be pitching my tent. *Speak to me*, I pleaded. But I kept riding as I was being ignored by the places I was passing. The darkness and exhaustion finally won out.

I fell off the bike.

"Fuck this!" I mumbled exhausted, dismounting The Beast. "This will have to do!"

I started pitching the tent on semi-flat rough ground, even though it was close to the road, only half-ass hidden behind tall pines. My aching, sweaty body crawled into the tent. My head felt heavy, and I knew I was dehydrated. As my sweat-soaked clothes began to chill, I used the last of my energy blowing into the pad, praying it would hold air for the night.

Dinner was a half of a bag of crumbled salt and vinegar chips. When the chips were gone, I licked my salty fingers and then ripped the bag open and licked the grease and salt and acid from inside the slick bag until it was shiny clean. Rolling onto my back, relieving the weight off my elbows, I gathered the last of my energy to send a text via satellite to Jim and the kids.

All dirt and loving it! I had ridden fifty-five miles and climbed 5,364 ft in ten hours and forty-two minutes. Salt and vinegar chips for dinner. A spectacular day finished riding with a full moon.

It was my first camp in Mexico. Sleeping on the side of the road by myself in the tent was definitely unnerving. I was pushing negative thoughts and fear out of my mind. I repeated my mantra: "I am not afraid! I am not afraid!" I was hoping no one could see me but the invisible spirits of the ancestors who were watching over me.

I closed my eyes. I was done. Listening to an owl hooting nearby was comforting, and I drifted off. They heard me! I was safe!

I woke up in the middle of the night with my pad completely deflated, leaving me on the cold, hard ground. A tiny pinecone poked me in the ribs, a small rock jabbed my bony hip, and another one protruded into my shoulder. My whole arm was numb.

It was 1:17 a.m., and I was wide awake. Moaning, I rolled off the pad. Blowing slowly into the cold black plastic valve, I breathed in and rested. I counted. Okay, just three more blows. Good enough! Rolling back onto the soft pad felt luxurious. I was back in dreamland fighting dragons. A few hours later, I woke up freezing, inflated the pad again, and waited for the first rays of the sun to penetrate the gray dawn. I hoped the sun would cast slivers of warmth onto my aching muscles through the paper-thin walls of the tent.

Maybe I was too old for this. Every part of me hurt. All this pushing my bike so many endless hours a day, sleeping on the hard ground, freezing all night, my leg cramping constantly.

Feeling unusually sorry for myself, I peeled the wrapper off a protein bar, snuggling under the quilt that was rated for much warmer nights. I was in Mexico. When were these nights going to get warmer, damnit? The gooey remains of the food bar stuck to my teeth and threatened to choke me. I had twenty-two miles left to go to *ejido* (communally owned) Sierra Juarez, a small community just before the town of Ojos Negros. I only had a half bottle of water left. None could be wasted.

Arriving at the ejido after a few hours, I stopped in the first store I passed to get a bottle of water and chocolate milk to help me recover from the grueling ride. I sat on the concrete steps next to my bike, leaned against the wall, closed my eyes, and drank. The cool water flowed through the entire twenty-five feet of my intestines. It was glorious to sense water entering every dehydrated cell. I made myself a promise to carry plenty of water and refill at every opportunity I had.

—NINETEEN—
Chupacabra

Maria, these walls were not meant to shut out problems.
You have to face them. You have to live the life you were
born to live.
—Mother Abbess from *The Sound of Music*

It was Thursday, October 25. I was in a cheap motel, fifteen dollars cheap, so cheap it was almost free. I was forced awake early, still in a daze, and wanted to sleep more as roosters screeched for warmth, begging the sun to rise. Dogs barked and played in the early dawn, and long-haul truckers fired up their big aging diesels for another day between the painted white lines. The din blasted right through my earplugs, and I reluctantly started packing my gear, which had mysteriously scattered itself around the room. The night before, I'd washed my riding shorts in the sink. They were still damp as I put them on, and chills darted through my aching body. I deflated my air mattress, which I'd tried to fix in the shower. I had found a couple of holes and tried to patch them with whatever I could find, but by morning, the mattress was limp again. Before departing, I tried to locate more holes by blowing up and dipping the unruly pad into the tiny bathroom sink, looking for bubbles to betray the leaks. It was like wrestling a giant crocodile. It did not, however, make me feel like

184

an Amazon warrior. I gave up, rolled the pad into its small stuff sack, and put it away, hoping that it would fix itself while I rode. I headed out at first light into the coolness of the morning.

The road took me out of Ojos Negro along green fields of produce waiting to be picked by low-paid migrant workers and trucked across the border to supermarkets across the US. Soon, I left the flat valley and started climbing at an even pace. Just a bit after noon I stopped at what I believed might be close to the highest point for the day. I found relief from the hot sun under a huge tree. A gentle, cooling breeze felt like a whisper in my face. As I took a pee, a deer ran no more than twenty feet from me. I started humming the tune from *The Sound of Music*, one of my favorite movies:

"(Do!), doe, a deer, a female deer,
(Re!) ray, a drop of golden sun. . . ."

We sang that song and others from the movie so many times when the kids were little. I played Maria, which is my baptized name. But how does one solve a problem like me? No one has been able to tell me that yet.

As I shoveled in some leftover pizza, I paused to take long sips of warm water. I was determined to do better at managing my water needs. I could not afford to run out of water riding so many miles a day. Afternoon temperatures were in the nineties.

And that's when it hit me—the real reason why I had hit the road in the first place, the thing I'd been dreaming about since I was a little girl: I was doing this! I was out here all by myself, loving the solitude. As tired as I was, moments like this made me feel more and more alive.

I pined for the chance to linger there—to pretend I was reclining against one of my grandfather's apple trees, a book of poetry in my hand and nowhere to be. I knew I would stay idle too long if I let myself. And then loneliness might overcome me. I needed to get my ass back on the bike. The day wasn't over yet, and as Jim would say, "We are burning daylight!" Yet, I hated to leave this wondrous place, asking myself why I was rushing. Rushing, rushing, like we do every day until life itself rushes past us, leaving us to wonder why the time flew by so quickly. Days and years go by, and we fail to stop and notice things we can only see if we slow down, pause and ponder the meaning of it all. At least for a bit. We owe that to ourselves.

The descent was steep and the road eroded, so I walked the bike over the roughest parts. There was no point taking the risk of falling and getting hurt way out there. I wondered how I would be rescued. Would I send an SOS through my Garmin InReach? Whom would they notify? The army? Would they send a helicopter? I wanted to know, but I really hoped I didn't need to use the SOS service. Whoever was dispatched, it would take them a long time to arrive at this remote and inhospitable place. I could die before they arrived. How ironic would that be?

Out in the distance, I saw palm trees and buildings. It looked like an abandoned ranch, but when I reached it, a few cows clumsily got up and scattered. An old pickup sat by a humble building. In America, there'd be no way that truck could possibly run, but Mexican people have amazing and creative skills to keep old vehicles chugging along. Necessity is the mother of creativity and reinvention.

The dirt road stretched to the horizon. It crossed mountain after mountain. I finally reached the valley of Uruapan, and I might as well have arrived in Tuscany. The area known for vineyards stretched into the hills on both sides of the valley. I rode on dirt through the village of very humble houses with neat little yards, dirt swept, flowers planted in tin cans. Somewhere along the way, I missed a sign that might have pointed to the hot springs where I planned to camp for the night. Even so, I stopped at a small convenience store with TECATE painted in bold letters and celebrated with a cold beer, then continued to Santo Thomas, where I knew there was a restaurant and a campground along the main road. After a day of solitude in the mountains, it was shocking to be back on busy Transpeninsular Highway 1 (also referred to as Mex 1), even if only for a few miles. I looked forward to waking up and riding along the coast, seeing the Pacific Ocean for the first time on my trip.

Gooood morning, legs! I practically sang to myself. I hadn't been this happy in a long time. I wanted the feeling to last forever.

It was Friday, October 26, my twenty-ninth straight day on the bike, and the climb out of Santo Tomas was as steep as promised. My legs were still tired after riding through rugged, challenging terrain the day before, and my muscles, heavy as lead, started burning and cramping.

I passed beautiful, lush vineyards lined in organized rows like soldiers standing at attention. Horses grazed lazily, their nostrils flaring in my direction. I imagined how pleasant it would be to finish this journey atop one of them. My heavy breathing matched the rhythm of every rotation of my pedals, and I rode in the lowest gear, often looking for one that was lower and not finding it. Sections of deep sand threatened to suck me up or throw me off The Beast.

The mood of the Pacific reached me way before I could see it. It smelled sharp and briny as my face was covered in mist carried by a timeless sea breeze. My bike made plenty of noise as it bounced along the rocky road, but I could hear a thunderous rumble coming closer. I rounded the corner, and the great vastness of the ocean greeted my whole body. Whitecaps rolled before me, the waves stretching endlessly in each direction, rushing toward the shore. A midmorning fog receded to the horizon. This was the grand Pacific I'd been waiting for!

After a steep descent that seemed to rattle loose my fillings, my hands cramping from squeezing the brakes, I reached a deserted fishing camp neatly tucked in the corner of a sandy bay. Gulls and frigates circled above looking for food. I snacked on avocado and nuts while my mind wandered freely. I watched a solitary gull gliding on the wind. Jonathan Livingston Seagull, learning the secrets of life by flying solo. I knew him.

The energy of the waves crashing on the beach vibrated through my body. Water. It's where all life begins. I listened to the ocean whispering promises to me. So many stories are born from the sea. Where does mine fit in?

The Pacific Ocean is the largest water mass on this planet of ours, covering more than 30 percent of Earth's surface. And yet it is also just a string of billions of water molecules, billions of water droplets, each one of them representing the sum of it all. Every wave ending on the shore and rushing back home is a promise of a new beginning. Somewhere in there is my story—my beginning and my end. Sitting on its shores, I felt the tremendous pull of this energy.

As much as I wanted to camp in this sandy beach cove, it seemed way too early in the day. I reluctantly kept riding. Just a bit farther down the road, I passed a sign for Rancho Tampico with big, bold letters above it saying PREAKUCION CHUPACABRAS!

The word *chupacabra* can literally be translated as "goat-sucker," a little factoid I just love. They are a legendary creature known in many parts of the Americas, said to suck the blood of farm animals. Jim has always liked the sound of the word *chupacabra*. When the kids were younger, he would repeat it over and over in a deep growling voice to scare them. They would just look at him laughing. I snapped a photo of the sign for Jim so I could send it to him when I had a signal. The road was leading me along the rugged Pacific coast to the town of ejido Eréndira. It was an active fishing community, and I found a restaurant overlooking the ocean, where I had my first Mexican fish taco meal.

I have always felt at home by the sea. My parents have a small house on the Croatian island of Šipan. With a population of less than five hundred, the island is part of a small archipelago stretching northwest of Dubrovnik in the Adriatic Sea. Quaint fishing villages, olive groves, rolling hilltops embellished with fragrant pine trees, and churches perched on top of the hills dating back to medieval times are all a natural setting for a romantic novel or, perhaps, a murder mystery. Vineyards produce delicious wines, and there are numerous fig trees and citrus groves. When I was a teenager, my family would spend summers there. If we were lucky, my brother and I would be invited to go fishing with the locals for the night. We would watch, spellbound, as they cast their nets and shined big lights into the depths of the ocean. Excitement ran high. The head fisherman would yell instructions, often cursing at the others. The boats moved expertly, swiftly closing the gaps in the nets, trapping a school of fish.

As a girl, I was instructed to sit down in the bow of the boat and stay out of the way, quiet and invisible. I was reminded over and over that I was lucky to even be on the boat. I was there only because the son of one of the fishermen had a crush on me, which allowed me to get around the superstitions about the female half of the human race.

"Women bring bad luck!" I had been told by the crusty old guys.

If the catch was good, laughter and singing followed. Muttering and blaming a woman came if the catch was poor. We'd sit around sorting fish by size and type into crates as the boat puttered into the night toward home. Returning to the village at dawn, I would board the six o'clock ferry to help sell the fish at the market in Dubrovnik. Once I was left alone at the stall while Vijeko went to run errands. No one stopped to buy my fish. "What is wrong?" I wondered. Then a man finally stopped, smoking the obligatory cigarette, a rolled-up newspaper tucked under his armpit.

"*Od dakle ova riba?*" He was pointing at the fish with his paper, asking who caught it.

"*Vijeko's from Sudurad.*" I answered shyly in my best Croatian, trying to imitate the local Dalmatian accent, hoping he wouldn't notice I was from Slovenia.

"*A kdje je ulovio?*" He wanted to know where the fish was caught.

"*Na jugu od Mljeta.*" Somewhere south of Island Mljet was the best description I could give with my limited knowledge of the region, especially since we were out fishing at night, and I had no clue where we were. Local fishermen were intimate with every nook and cranny of the islands by fishing with their fathers and their father's fathers since they were able to walk.

"*Onda daj mi kilo!*" In that case, give me one kilo, the man said, finally recognizing the name of the fisherman.

I then realized no one wanted to buy fish from someone who wasn't a local, especially a blonde sixteen-year-old foreign girl in red Adidas shorts and a crisp white tank top who stood out like a sore thumb from the other women and men in black aprons. I did not fit in, as much as I wanted to. My father kept a vigilant watch over me in those years. He was terrified that any summer romance with local boys would become too serious.

"You would never fit in here," he often lectured me. "It's fun for the summer, but life on the island is not for a girl like you. You would never feel at home here, and you'll always be an outsider, a foreigner."

"I like it here, Dad," I would try to explain. "Life is simple, unspoiled and beautiful."

"You see it that way now; it's a romantic vision of the place. But spend a year or two here, taking care of your babies and never leaving the island, and you'll think differently. What are you going to do here?"

"I could write books," I said optimistically. "There are so many interesting stories here."

"You could, but you need an education and your own life experiences for that first," My dad wisely answered. "Go spread your wings. This island will always be here for you."

Sitting in the Mexican restaurant, my nostalgia for life on our island returned. I was older if not wiser, and surely more experienced. The idea of living on Šipan and writing wasn't so farfetched anymore. Quietly, I savored the moment.

I continued riding along the coast as the waves crashed onto the rocky shore, throwing high plumes of foam several feet into the air.

Once the road left the ocean, it became eroded with impossibly deep ruts and washpan rollers from years of the Baja 1000. It is one of the most prestigious off-road races in the world and has been running for more than fifty years. I now understood why they change the roads they ride on every year. They were practically impassable after race cars, motorcycles, trucks, ATVs, and buggies carved deep ruts into them.

I had phone service and talked with Mateja for a while. That revived me a bit, as I was getting fatigued. As usual, she was upbeat and encouraging. With all she's gone through during and after her accident, her resilience was my inspiration. She never looked back, made any excuses, or held any grudges. She simply moved on and adapted. She was able to get out of her wheelchair, and although she wouldn't be running anytime soon, she was walking again. Our conversation distracted me as I struggled in and out of eroded canyons. I had anticipated riding on twenty-six miles of smooth, flat road, which would allow me to coast into town. "It's always farther than it looks. It's always taller than it looks. And it's always harder than it looks," My childhood hero, Reinhold Messner reminded me. I was following my dream, conceived as this strong man—a man taller than the tallest mountain on Earth, with eyes bluer than the bluest lake—shook my tiny hand. This was my healing journey, a journey to claim back my life. I needed to prove to myself, my family, and my friends that I would not be defeated by life, which had challenged me beyond my imagination.

I arrived at the town of Colonet by headlamp. I passed no motel or campground and realized I should have camped somewhere along the coast, even though it meant canned tuna for dinner again. I'd passed so many beautiful small coves but chickened out on camping alone. I also knew that Jim would prefer if I stayed in a motel, especially when I was closer to the towns, and I agreed with him. I passed many crudely built structures on the outskirts of town. They had no lights. Some had small fires built in front of them. The town stretched along both sides of the highway. I made some inquiries about a motel and was told I had to ride a couple miles north of town on the main road, still busy with cars and trucks. I had no choice. Reluctantly I started riding on the main road, praying loudly to The Beast and myself. The road climbed, had no shoulder, and the sky was dark as coal. The trucks drove fast, and every time one whizzed by, the bike swayed like a tiny boat on a turbulent sea.

I dismounted the bike to walk so I could stay as far off the pavement as much as possible, trying not to roll into the ditch. I prayed that the flashing red light on the back of my bike was bright enough for drivers to see. I knew Jim was tracking me back home. He did so every night until I could call him or send him a text. He was able to see that I was on the side of the highway, and I knew he was worried.

It seemed like an eternity, but I finally reached the Hotel Paradisio, and at that moment, it lived up to its name. I was filthy and exhausted, but incredibly relieved that I had arrived unscathed.

I leaned my dusty bike against a post, and a sliding door opened into a dimly lit hotel lobby with a shiny marble floor. My bike shoes clunked loudly and echoed in the quiet space.

"*Hola!*" I called into the abyss. Nothing. "*¿Con permiso?*" I called again, and the thought of just camping in the lobby on the couch crossed my mind. The night manager finally came from the direction of the kitchen. I gladly exchanged my credit card for a room key. I clunked out of the lobby and rolled the bike into the room on the ground floor. I shut the door, and the privacy of the room felt like a glorious palace. I quickly sent Jim a message that I had arrived safely at a hotel. It was after ten o'clock, and the restaurant, of course, was closed, but the manager sent a quesadilla and a cold Corona to my room. There was a lime wedge wrapped in a napkin. It was a feast. A shower and a clean, soft bed never felt better. Falling into bed naked and exhausted, I felt almost human again. It was a home away from home. I wrote a bit, just to capture a few details from the day, but quickly grew tired. I stretched out wide in the king-size bed. The crisp, cool, white sheets soothed my skin, soft from the soapy shower and cheap fragrant body lotion, compliments of the hotel. I wedged my body between pillows soft as a newborn puppy and drifted into a peaceful sleep.

As American gospel choirs sing, day by day, mile by mile, I was getting healed.

–TWENTY–
Am I Lost?

I'm not lost for I know where I am. But, however,
where I am may be lost.
—*Winnie-the-Pooh*, A.A. Milne

Saturday, October 27, marked a month from when I left home. No matter how I measured it, the previous day had wiped me out: sixty miles, more than 3,000 feet of climbing, and riding on rutted dirt roads to finally arrive safely at a hotel in blackness. I had been on the bike, my only companion, for a long and grueling time. Exhaustion was starting to get to me. I thought again of Reinhold Messner, whose provocative question came back to me: "So, is man born to go alone? To *go* alone at times, yes, but not to *be* alone." At that moment I couldn't find comfort in his words.

As much as I craved solitude on the outset of this trip, I had never been alone for so long. Yes, there was joy in being alone, but there wasn't any joy in not being able to share both fear and beautiful moments. Deep down I feared that I was getting used to being by myself and liking it. I was afraid to admit to myself that I was glad Jim hadn't come along on the trip. I enjoyed the pace of being a loner, leaving whenever I felt like, stopping in places that felt right to me without having to compromise with someone else. There was no one to complain to about how difficult the riding was, and that felt good. In solitude, I found a very different kind of strength, one I'd never experienced. I was purging poisons from my body and mind. I was cultivating the soil in which fresh seeds of life could be planted again. And for that, I needed to be alone, as painful or as lonely as it sometimes felt.

For breakfast, I pulled over where the road overlooked numerous fields. I unwrapped a protein bar and a stick of string cheese. I'd found the cheese stuffed in a bag that holds my bike tools, a leftover gift from the Mexican family in California. Riding along, I passed people walking to work the fields. They all had big smiles on their faces. When I waved to them, they always waved back. Throughout my trip I'd found that people everywhere just want to live happy, productive, and meaningful lives. They want to work so they can have a place they can call home, provide for their families, and send their kids to school.

Even so, I could never really let my guard down completely.

I stopped to resupply at ejido Benito Suarez. A toothless but very friendly guy admired my bike.

"How much does this bike cost?" he asked, staring at the bike and everything on it.

"Oh, I don't know. Not that much. I forget," I answered lamely, not being able to make up something more clever in my limited Spanish.

"I have a bike at home. I can go get it and ride with you into the mountains. It's a long and steep road, and a long way to Rancho Coyote from this side."

"Oh no, that's okay, I ride slow. I have my maps." I pointed to my Garmin navigation device on my bike. "This will show me the way."

I hopped on the bike and rode off, fast. Much faster than I wanted to. He seemed like a nice enough guy, but the fact was, I was a woman

traveling alone and uncomfortable to have a stranger for a companion. I kept turning around, making sure he wasn't following me.

Soon I was in remote canyons crossing water in arroyos that
reached over my knees. These dry creeks or washes fill with water after
heavy rains, causing flash flooding, and the roads leading through
often change. I was suddenly following the wrong one, and the mistake wasted a precious hour. The road climbed toward the high pass I
had to cross before reaching Rancho Coyote where, I assumed, a cold
beer would be waiting for me. Salvador Felipe Meling Johnson had
established el Coyote Rancho four generations prior. Although they
still export cattle to Mexico's mainland, it is now open to the public,
and they offer cabins, camping, fishing, hunting, and ecotours to vis-
itors from all over the world. The area is also known worldwide for
endless dirt-biking trails.

I felt safest when I was really far out and away from towns.
When I was confident that the guy was not following me, I sat
down on a rock to have a snack and water and rest. I loved listening to the wind and the birds, and that was about all there was
out there until looking closer, I became more intimate with my
surroundings. Then I noticed coyotes, bunnies, snakes, and all
kinds of insects crawling over rocks. If you looked more carefully,
the rocks hid delicate flowers as transparent as a thin sheet of ice.
They bloomed as soon as rain touched them. I kicked a rock, and
an almost translucent scorpion darted in my direction. I jumped
up and got back on my bike.

I entered a remote canyon road, and a pickup and a 4x4 SUV
passed me. It looked to me like the locals were taking tourists hunting. It was scorching hot, and I was riding only in my shorts and
sports bra. As the trucks passed, I got inquisitive stares by the men
sitting in both vehicles that made me feel uneasy. Then the road

started climbing, and it rose as steep as any I had been on. At least, that's how it felt whenever I huffed and puffed and pushed and sometimes dragged The Beast with all my gear. Loose rock and smooth slabs of granite prevented me from riding much of it, so I pushed The Beast and begged it to cooperate. It didn't. The going was slow!

Suddenly, my digital map disappeared. There was no purple line, no arrows, no nothing—just a blank, gray screen staring back at me. I could not have possibly gone wrong anywhere! I'd already been climbing this damn road for two hours! I didn't recall passing any other dirt roads. I kept going with a twisting feeling in my gut until I finally reached the top. Was I on the right pass? Was I lost? I sat down on a rock and reset the Garmin by turning it off for a few seconds, then, with acid rising to my throat from my stomach, turning it back on. It took time recalculating. I held my breath. The map showed up, and my dot was on the purple line right where I was supposed to be. I let out a huge sigh of relief.

I could finally enjoy a snack and some water. The SUV that had passed me a few hours before returned from around the mountain. It turned out the people traveling in it weren't hunters at all. They stopped, and we chatted in my best possible Spanish. A professor from Ensenada was leading a group of scholars from Japan to look for the marmot migration. Who would have thought? Again, I had made an assumption based on looks alone. But as Thoreau says in *Walden*, "It is never too late to give up our prejudices." And what is the purpose of travel, but to do just that!

"When we travel," says my dear friend Tom O'Neil, "we expand our minds. It is a simple way to make the world a better place, by understanding other cultures, especially when we immerse ourselves in them on a deeper level."

Mark Twain also tells us, "Broad, wholesome, charitable views of men and things cannot be acquired by vegetating in one little corner of the earth all one's lifetime."

As much as I'd traveled all my life, I still had to be reminded of that!

This long ride was helping me understand more and more about myself. I was starting to see more clearly. I noticed small details around me that would otherwise have passed by. My sense of smell was sharper. It was as if I could sense things around me with the surface of my skin. I could feel things around me with my eyes closed. I felt as if I were returning into the kingdom of a wild woman and natural creatures that couldn't be tamed.

My former husband gave me the book *Women Who Run With The Wolves* by Clarrisa Pinkola Estés in the hope that it might satisfy my wild nature. But instead of appeasing me, this wild woman archetype gave me courage to look deeper within myself and acknowledge something I had been given at birth. It revealed the driving forces within me I'd been trying to understand. I had an adventurous spirit, yet I craved stability and security. And I never understood that it was okay to seek a balance of both. I didn't know how to stand up for myself.

Tom was fifteen years my senior, and in the beginning of our marriage, he represented the father figure I had desperately needed. But I grew into a woman who didn't want to compromise my fundamental beliefs. There was a false sense of freedom as long as I stayed within the confines of his territory. He always knew better because he was older, wiser, more educated. I looked up to him like I looked up to my older brother and my father. But I started to feel trapped in a world I'd helped create. As I read, I highlighted many paragraphs like: *They marry while they are naive about predators, and they choose someone who is destructive to their lives. They are determined to "cure" that person with love.* I've always believed in love but didn't actually know what love was. I was consumed by the realization of what our relationship had become. It was as if the words I was reading had been written for me.

Do what I say, and I will love you was the message I received. And, on the other hand, I will do whatever I want, including pursuing other women if I so wish.

I married young because I got pregnant, but I also wanted to make things work. I loved my children. And I compromised. Instead of living freely, I began living falsely. Estés's words rang louder in my ears. At one point in the book, she wrote: "There is a way out of all this, but one must have a key."

In the end, it turned out that my key was divorce. It took years after the trust was broken, the very foundation of a healthy relationship, to have the courage to turn the key and unlock the door. This ride was demanding a different kind of courage—transformational and healing—pulled from depths I did not know I possessed.

Getting up from the rock, I stretched my arms toward the sky and looked around. In every direction I saw nothing but brown rocks and mountains. It seemed as if I were standing on the surface of Mars. I felt like a powerful queen in my own universe, even though it was composed of nothing but dirt and rock. The road disappeared before me. I saw no end to it. I took a deep breath and exhaled all the air from my lungs. It made me dizzy. I was drunk on freedom.

The Beast and I peddled up and down miles and miles of the challenging, rough, rocky trail. The shadows grew longer as the day waned, and the temperature dropped, which felt really nice. I got a text from Jim, who was following my progress.

"It looks like you have three miles to go!"

"Yes!" I replied by pushing a preset message function on my InReach.

And then, about another hour later: "You can make it!"

At the moment, I needed that encouragement so desperately. Jim was able to see how long it was taking me to cover a short distance. The trail was steep, and progress was painfully slow. It seemed as if I were standing still. Would I ever reach the rancho? Most of the time I was pushing The Beast up impossibly steep, rocky hills, breathing hard and cursing when I slid backward. I developed a technique: push, squeeze the brakes, and take a step; push, squeeze the brakes, and take a step. Coyotes howled at the darkening sky, and God knows what else was out there at this late hour. I had a creepy feeling I was being followed. With the night rapidly descending, my fears grew just as quickly. I was mentally preparing to pitch my tent behind one of the giant granite boulders, when yet another text buzzed through my device. "You are almost there."

"Thank you, Jim," I whispered with relief. "Yes" I sent a preset message button for the second time back to Jim and pushed on with a new burst of energy.

The last half a mile before el Coyote Rancho, I was led by another owl. It landed on the trail in front of me, flew away when I caught up with it, and landed about twenty feet away. It went like that until I reached the gate to the rancho. I had always thought a white mountain goat was my spirit animal. The goat spirit symbolizes a sense of independence and reminded me to look up and move forward. My father and my mother also often compared me to a mountain goat when they described my stubborn self, usually when they were frustrated with me. More often than not, it would make me feel bad and guilty. Being stubborn is not necessarily looked upon as an endearing quality. But maybe this owl, which was showing me the way, was my true spirit animal. An owl represents a deep connection with wisdom, good judgment, and knowledge. It has sharp vision and keen observation. It possesses insight and intuition. I liked this version of me. Now I think my goat spirit animal has evolved into an owl. I just needed to be a goat first, before I turned into a wise old owl. I had developed sharp vision to help me see beyond the masks people wear. Riding my bike alone in those remote and formidable places, I was shedding my own mask.

I untied the rope holding the barbed-wire fence and felt as if I were opening the door to the safe home I'd been searching for. The darkness pushed on me like a blanket, and I had no idea where to go. As I passed a dark trailer, a truck came down the hill driven by a ranch hand who pointed me toward the main house. Alfredo, who runs the place, directed me to a spot under a large tree to set up camp. I quickly sent another preset message to Jim: "Stopping for the night. All is well." While I was setting up the tent, Alfredo's beautiful young wife, Carla, brought me three bean burritos and a cold Tecate. I was so grateful, as I ate the meal. I soon fell asleep without brushing my teeth. I was warm enough and only had to inflate my pad three times during the night.

I awoke to a symphony of cows, sheep, and birds. I inflated the pad one last time and enjoyed the harmony of the ranch in the comfort of my tent before I saw it. As I was making coffee, a guy walked toward me with a chair in his hands. Three sheep followed him like little puppies.

I could tell he was a gringo.

Mike and his wife Nannette had lived in Vicente Guerrero for twenty-seven years. Mike lived in a trailer on the rancho pretty much full-time, and Nannette joined him on weekends. He was seventy-five when I met him. He used to install solar power systems in the area. He and I immediately connected as we philosophized about life. He showed me a logbook of riders who had come through on the Baja Divide. Many people skip this section because it's so strenuous, so I was only the twenty-fourth person to sign the book over the last two years. I was also the oldest solo woman by far. I allowed myself to feel just a tad proud.

After a hot shower that rinsed away the dirt of the road, I returned to camp to find a plate piled with three eggs, two potatoes, a banana, and two granola bars. I decided that the ranch would be an excellent place for my first day of rest in over a month. Mike's generosity made it possible for me to stay an extra day. And what a breakfast and lunch that made! I flavored it up with spices I had from the Louisiana Spiceman.

I was in heaven sitting under the tree. Mike fixed my sleeping pad, and I had time to do absolutely nothing at all. Eventually I tended to a few things on my bike, fixed my broken reading glasses with dental floss, read, planned for the next leg of my trip, and wrote. After exploring the ranch, I even took a nap. Mike said he always tinkers with things. I thought he was like a mad scientist who could fix just about anything. I gave him a battery charger pack I'd found along the trail the previous day, and the man was like a kid at Christmas. I'm sure he was able to fix it.

Rancho El Coyote lies on a plateau at three thousand feet above sea level. The surrounding mountains make up the Sierra San Pedro Martir range and reach higher than ten thousand feet. They are breathtaking monuments of splendor. If you are lucky enough, you can see a giant condor that has been reintroduced as well as pumas, bobcats, and bighorn sheep called cimarron. In winter it often snows in the peaks and sometimes even at the ranch. Massive white granite boulders of all shapes make your imagination run wild as you ride by them, especially in the evening light when shadows run long, and the sky is colored red. I was a white mountain goat with an owl perched on its head, standing on top of the largest boulder. I was the fairy queen Titania ruling over my own kin.

—TWENTY-ONE—
The Beauty in Being Alone

O please, O please, Come out and play.
For we have not come here to take prisoners
Or to confine our wondrous spirits,
But to experience ever and ever more deeply
Our divine courage, freedom, and Light!
—Hafiz, Sufi poet

On Monday, October 29, my day at the ranch was passing way too quickly. Later in the afternoon, Nanette came over and got right into it.

"Why are you riding? I mean, we see young people coming through, mostly couples, or groups, or guys who ride alone, but never women, especially older women like you. You seem different. I mean, how old are you anyway?"

"Fifty-four." This time my age came out easily. I felt a deep sense of pride in saying it.

"Oh, I actually thought you were more like in your forties."

"Oh? Well, thanks for that!" I said with a smile on my face. "It's a good question, Nanette. I think I'm trying to figure that out myself."

"People are usually running away from things when they do something like this," she observed.

I thought about that for a moment and then responded, "Most people would think I'm running away from all the stuff that happened to me, but it's more than that. It's more like I'm running toward something new. I guess I'm on some sort of a quest to reinvent myself."

I contemplated further.

"Being on this extended bike ride allows me to detach myself from all my problems. It is forcing me to just focus on immediate issues I need to deal with, like food, water, riding, and looking for a place to sleep. Like climbing a big mountain, it is survival in its purest form."

"I know you might not want to talk about it, but what *did* happen to you?"

I told her what the past two years had wrought. Then I paused, and we both just sat in silence looking at the grazing sheep. The ranch dog came and placed his head in my lap. I spoke up again.

"I had a need to get away from it all. I don't know if my cancer will come back. I don't know how my husband's disease will progress, or how much time we have to do the things we want to do. I feel as if this is my last window of opportunity to do something I've always wanted to do."

She nodded. "Well, none of us knows what the future will bring, especially at our age," she said. "But not everyone goes out to challenge themselves quite like this. Is it fun?"

"*Fun* is a strong word." I laughed. "No, a lot of the time it's not fun. I don't think it's supposed to be, either. We don't necessarily find a deeper meaning about life by just doing what's easy or fun. That comes by challenging ourselves beyond what we think we are capable of."

"It sounds hard, painful. I'd be pretty scared out there by myself, especially at night. Did you know there were pumas out here?"

"I didn't know that until Alfredo warned me about them when I went up to talk to him and pay for my camp. I am glad I didn't, especially last night when I was going through these last canyons at dusk."

"Yes, dusk and dawn is when they are most active and hunting."

"Should I worry?"

"They hunt for goats. It's not going to do you any good to worry anyway. Just stay alert, keep a whistle and pepper spray close at hand."

She encouraged me to talk further about my trip. I found myself speaking as much to myself as to her.

"I am definitely challenged every day. I've never done anything like this before. I've climbed a lot of mountains in my life. I know the feeling when you think you can't go one step farther, and then you make it to the top. You look around, and there's that profound feeling of accomplishment when you realize, This is why I am doing this! No one did it for me. I've earned it myself. But this ride? This is different. I'm connecting all the dots in my confusing and often painful life. I have a lot of time to think and process things while I ride. Trying to somehow make sense of it, understand why all these things are happening to me. I am not sure I can ever understand it all, but I've asked not to be tested any more after every terrible event I've gone through. Those are the times I've prayed to God, hoping desperately for his or her existence, wishing I believed."

I paused.

"I prayed to the powers of the Great Universe, 'No more please, I can't take it anymore.' The irony is, though, that now I am testing *myself*. I am pushing myself harder than I've ever been pushed."

"Do you ever cry?" she asked.

"I don't think I've cried on this whole trip because it was physically difficult or because I was sad or hurt or scared. I've cried when I worry about my husband or when I miss him. I've cried when I've been touched deeply by people I've met along the way. Those are good, healing tears. Then I keep moving, and I feel better. In movement, surrounded by nature, I feel I am most alive."

All these thoughts seemed to suddenly come together at that precise moment and finally made sense to me.

"I also feel like I finally have control over my own actions," I said. "I had no control over all the poking and probing, cutting into my body, x-rays, MRIs, radiation, poisonous chemicals that were supposed to heal me, yet were the opposite of what I thought were my beliefs about healing."

Another long pause. "I had to surrender to an onslaught of contradictions."

We both sat in silence for a long time, immersed in our own thoughts. A quiet understanding settled between us. The three pet sheep peacefully grazed on the grass around us. I watched them, pondering how sheep don't have to worry about all the stuff we humans do. Being a sheep would be so much simpler.

Nanette invited me to dinner. Mike went to bed early. She cooked rice and beans in a solar oven Mike had built. We seasoned the meal with the spices from my Spiceman friend. I left the bag of spices for Nannette and Mike. I wished I could repay them with more, but it was all I had left.

Mike had lent me a sleeping pad while he was fixing mine, so I had a restful night. In the morning, I reluctantly packed to leave the unique oasis. My body and my mind had received much-needed rest. I bid goodbye to Mike and Nannette and promised to stay in touch. Nannette waved and called after me, "I will come and find you in La Ventana!" Rancho El Coyote was yet another place I'd like to return for a visit with Jim. I hope that when I finally do, Mike and Nannette will still be there.

The dirt road led me along beautiful boulder hills five miles toward Rancho Meling. I wished I could ride like that forever! I stopped to snack on a precious banana I'd been saving, but it must have jumped off the bike going over a bump somewhere on that downhill road. Crossing the creek in the arroyo, the trail led me away from the ranch, and then steep hills started one after another for more than five miles. I had to walk and push the bike with my already perfected technique of pushing, then squeezing the brake before taking another step. I could see why older people who live alone talk to themselves, their pets, or their bikes, for that matter. I felt like I was Don Quixote talking to his horse, Rocinante, during their trek. Like Quixote, I was awkward, past my prime, and engaged in a task beyond my capacities.

Still, I believed in the power of the quest.

At the end of thirty-four miles of steep climbing and riding over dry and desolate terrain, I was rewarded with a technically challenging but enjoyable drop into an arroyo that brought me to Vicente Guerrero. The Beast, equipped with front and rear shock absorbers, handled narrow, steep, and bumpy single-track superbly. That was my favorite technical downhill of the trip, until I dove headfirst over the handlebars, feeling as if I were riding a bucking bronco. Arriving in town only mildly scratched after the crash, I stopped at FASS bike shop and dropped The Beast off for a spa treatment, which he needed after being on the road for more than a month. They cleaned and coated the chain with fresh, wax-based lube and replaced the rear brake pads. Salvador, the shop owner, snapped a photo of The Beast and me for his hall of fame wall, then directed me to a trail that would lead me on some single-track trail toward San Quintin.

On Tuesday, October 30, I arrived at San Quintin in the late afternoon. I found a fifteen-dollar motel called Chavez that was comfortable enough and looked safe. When I returned to the room after dinner across the street, truck after truck pulled in, and with them, lots of noise. Doors slammed behind call girls entering rooms. The motel was full, and TVs blared through paper-thin walls, mixing with screams and moans. The girls left with more slamming doors. I couldn't drown out the noise, even with double earplugs stuffed deep. Sleep was out of the question. I watched the local news about a caravan of people heading toward the US border. Some were walking, some were riding on the backs of trucks, while others drove in fully packed cars. When I finally dozed off, my dreams flooded with images of mothers and fathers holding onto their kids, running through the hot, dry desert, and babies crying when they were separated from their mothers. People fled their homes and hoped to find safety, but no one wanted them.

I woke up confused, distraught, and feeling guilty, knowing this was not just my nightmare but reality for so many people. It was a selfish act, running away from my own problems instead of helping others in need. I couldn't wait to get out of the busy, loud, agricultural town. I couldn't wait to get away from my own guilty thoughts.

I tried pushing my nightmares away by listening to a book on my phone. John Grisham's novel, *The Reckoning*, was as good a distraction as any. But I kept thinking about the suffering and how I was trying to shut other people's problems out of my mind. Will I ever be forgiven for that?

I rode through salt marshes toward three volcanoes framing the Bay of San Quintin. Near an abandoned, half-finished hotel, three black turkey vultures stood atop a crumbling wall with their majestic wings spread six feet wide as if waiting for me: "Guilty. Guilty. Guilty." Their guttural sounds followed me as I picked up the pace, not looking back.

Reaching my camp five miles before Nueva Odisea at lunchtime was just fine. After riding on firm salt flats, I switched to crawling speed for several miles on a deep sandy road. I pushed the bike through the heat of the day. Sand dunes separated me by a few hundred feet from the cool Pacific Ocean. Every time I tried to get across to the waterfront, where I was hoping the beach would be firmer to ride on, soft sand forced me to turn back and continue slogging through ankle-deep sand on the road. I had woken up for several days dreading the thought of getting on my bike. I'd been pushing myself too hard. So, I took time in the afternoon to sit on the beach and watch waves and shorebirds, cherishing the fact I had the whole beach and the ocean to myself. I took off my bike shoes and dipped my toes in the water. My feet dug into the silky, soft sand as wave after infinite wave seeped across blistered, sore toes, gently washing away days of pain. I reminded myself again that if I was not enjoying my time at least a little during this trip, it was not worth doing. I was aware I had a tough section ahead of me in remote high country where I'd have to carry all my food and water for several days. My body, and especially my mind, needed to be ready.

Before I was engulfed again in the darkness of the night, I wanted to feel the wonder of the air around me, notice the light as it changed from hot and bright to light pink to subtle blue, then misty gray at the edge of dusk. I wanted to experience the necessity of the moment, live on the edge of my abilities. For the time being, things went on in the world without me. They'd still be there when I got back. My fear was only how much I'd like it when I did return, the politics and all the things we believe need to be done, all the rushing, coming, and going without knowing what actually matters. Without noticing the magic and the beauty of everyday things like the way the morning light illuminates the leaf just right as you hurry by on your way to work. We are convinced we need so many material things, which in the end makes us prisoners of the lives we create. I missed my husband, family, and friends, but I knew they would be there when I returned, and we'd all be happily reunited.

For now, though, I traveled alone with my feelings and thoughts, and there was beauty in being alone. Like everyone else, I often tended to forget how to balance that fine line of being alone and feeling lonely, but I was learning.

—TWENTY-TWO—
Water Please

Even a fool learns something once it hits him.
—Homer, *Iliad*

Wednesday, 1 November, was *Dia de los Muertos*. The Day of the Dead is celebrated throughout Mexico, particularly in the central and southern regions. It is also recognized in other Catholic countries around the world. The multiday holiday focuses on gathering with family and friends to pray for and remember those who have died and to support their spiritual journey.

Slovenia is a predominantly Catholic country. Visiting the graves of family members was a big deal on the first day of November. My grandma would grow flowers all fall so they would be ready to take to our family plot in Ljubljana. She was always praying they would survive the frost and make it until the Day of the Dead when all the graves were tidied and decorated with flowers and candles. When we were kids, we had to dress in our finest clothes and walk solemnly behind our parents. Women, including my mother, hoped it would be cold enough to show off their mink and fox fur coats. My brother and I dreaded all that. My dad would roll his eyes in surrender. I remember my brother and I were quite young when we went shopping in Italy for new Levi jeans and jean jackets. We were so excited to get the groovy new clothes. It was the height of fashion then, and we knew we would be the coolest kids in town wearing those clothes. We begged our mother on our knees, and she finally gave in and allowed us to wear them for the special day. Boy, did my mother get in trouble for that! In the eyes of our grandmother, we looked like a couple of hooligans, and she made it known we were a big embarrassment to the family.

I remember the whole scene gave my father great pleasure. He considered dressing up properly to be unnecessary and conforming. Running an IBM education center, he had to wear a white shirt and tie to work every day and was not a fan of it. He found it very amusing that we talked my mother into breaking the rule. I think he secretly enjoyed messing with his mother-in-law. My grandmother grew up poor, third in a line of six sisters, and was orphaned at a very young age. Their mother died of consumption soon after she gave birth to her sixth daughter, Fini. Father Johan married their maid, and they produced another son. But tuberculosis would also claim the life of my great-grandfather only one year after the death of his first wife.

After they were orphaned, all the girls scattered to different homes to be raised separately. The oldest sister, Mary, who trained to be a seamstress, finally gathered her sisters under one roof. Somehow, with hard work, they survived. Nuns took in the youngest one, and she later became a sister in St. Valentine's order. My grandmother worked hard all her life. I now understand she didn't want people to think we were poor. How we dressed and how we behaved was of great importance to her. Wearing American style clothes on the Day of the Dead just wasn't right, in her mind.

Neither was pushing or shoving, nor walking on the edges of other gravestones as we proceeded through crowds to our family plot under the constant stern watch of our grandmother. Curbing the energy of our youth, we had to shake strangers' hands politely and listen again and again to how much we had grown in the past year.

Families maintained a strict unstated competition about whose plot looked more beautiful and more ostentatious. As kids, we lived for lighting the candles. The fire of life, remembering the dead. The best part of the day was the family gathering for a big lunch afterward: goulash soup with dumplings, grilled meats, potato salad, cabbage salad, vanilla crescent cookies, and potica—a traditional Slovenian walnut roll—were the reward for our good behavior at the graves. Finally, my dad could relax, loosen up his cravat, which he despised wearing on his non-working days, and enjoy a well-deserved beer.

In mainland Mexico, Dia de los Muertos is a colorful three-day celebration of life and death, where people wear colorful clothes, paint their faces, and dance in the street, especially at night. Graves are decorated with fresh-cut flowers of all colors, and the light from hundreds of candles illuminates the cemeteries. Here in this remote area of Baja desert, I saw none of that. I passed many graves decorated with a fantastic array of plastic flowers; they lasted longer and didn't need water, perfect for the hot desert.

In Nueva Odisea, I filled up on water and bought an apple, an egg, and some chocolate milk. The road started climbing away from the Pacific, and it soon came to beautiful slopes studded with boulders strewn about like randomly tossed coins. I liked it. I stopped for lunch at a beautiful vista point, looking down toward the Pacific. It was getting hot, and I was concerned that I didn't have enough water for this part of the ride. I knew I could survive by finding water in cacti. There were fruits I could eat. I was resourceful. I was returning to my optimistic, confident self, not considering that I could be fooling myself.

Arriving at the next plateau, I saw a growth of pitaya dulce cacti with large golf-ball-sized red fruit hanging off the many branches. I dismounted The Beast and took out my knife to cut off a piece of fruit that looked young and soft, thinking this had to be the perfect one. The flesh was soft pink and inviting, so I cut it open and bit into it. Suddenly my whole mouth, my tongue, and my gums were full of laser thin needles. I couldn't even close my mouth. I was gasping for air, waving my arms like two broken propellers. The needles were sticking in my lips as well, and all over my bike gloves, penetrating my fingers. Bad idea! First, I struggled to take off my gloves to find my tweezers in my first aid kit. I started the slow process of removing the hardly visible, fiberglass-like slivers from my fingers, lips, tongue, and gums. Many of them broke off, and I was hoping they would dissolve in time and not cause infection. I felt foolish, thinking I was so full of knowledge and confidence. My gloves were worthless. Humbled, I got back on my bike. My tongue kept searching inside my mouth, finding tiny bumps swelling everywhere.

I later learned that the fruit you are supposed to pick has to be dark red; the needles have to fall off if you just touch them, and the fruit has to snap off the branch without effort, with a light tap. That is how you know pitaya dulce fruit is ripe.

As the temperature neared a hundred degrees, I was down to two bottles of water with sixty miles to go. I finally crested the last summit, and the rough road started to descend. I was excited to go downhill when something started making a funny noise in the back of my bike. I ignored it, planning to deal with it when I stopped. It got louder and louder. I slowed down and found a water bottle holder mounted on the back barely hanging on by one zip tie. Miraculously, the water bottle was still in it. I'd been saving every drop of water, and this was my last full bottle.

The evening sky painted a magical rosy glow on the edge of the horizon, and I found myself surrounded by cirios and cardón cacti. The silhouettes of the mountain ridges and cacti of all different sizes and shapes were etched into the skyline. One singular mountain glowed bright gold, lit up by the setting sun. It looked as if I'd entered a fairytale. From afar, the cirios looked like giant smooth carrots with soft white tufts of flowers decorating the tops, like a toupee stuck on the head of an old man. As I rode closer, I noticed the trunks were covered with leaves and needles, which sprout profusely after it rains. Some cirios were thick, some thin, and some split into multiple trunks, either sticking up in different directions or curling back down to the earth, bowing before me to admit me into their solitary desert magic. No two alike, each possessed the personality of a slightly tipsy soldier standing next to the sergeant cardón, which had a uniformly straight thick trunk, often with two or more arms lifted next to the main body.

I felt as if I had abruptly landed on a different planet. I may not have known their language, but I felt welcome, so I returned their greeting, hollering out loud.

"Hola, amigos!" I yodeled.

I expected an echo like when I'd yodeled in the Alps as a girl, but the vast and arid desert swallowed my voice.

Suddenly the whole day's effort had paid off. Now I just had to find the right place to camp for the night. I passed a dry arroyo, and just up the hill from it stood a group of trees, a fire pit, and just enough light left to pitch the tent. I leaned The Beast against the tree and got tangled in the branches, which were covered by needles I hadn't noticed before. I pried my sleeve loose, but then my hair got caught by the same branch, and as I was trying to untangle my hair, I pricked my gloveless hands, and they started bleeding.

"Let me go!" I screamed at the tree and pulled away from it, finally freeing myself.

Resembling a madwoman possessed by evil spirits, I ran off into the desert, screaming. When I realized how stupid that was, I stopped, and gathered wood for the fire, and headed back to camp. The tent wasn't going to set itself up. The light was fading, and the desert was quickly cooling down. I built a small fire, and the process of doing something—anything—calmed me down. My soup cooked over the fire while I blew air into my mattress pad. One cup of water was my ration. I had to save what was left to ride the next sixty miles. Using my headlamp and my skewed reading glasses, I began removing fine needles from my gloves. My mouth and my lips were swollen and tender.

I let the fire die down to charcoal, which gave me plenty of warmth but allowed me enough darkness to watch the Milky Way stretching above me. Bright stars flickered, unspoiled by any ambient light, and I gave in to listening to the grand finale of the birds' symphony as they finished in unison before retiring for the night. It came in the form of the loudest crescendo I'd ever heard. Then in an instant, all was quiet. The sky was blood red, and I was bloody tired. My rice noodle soup was overcooked, the noodles all soggy and clumped together. I forced myself to eat it anyway. It was the only source of calories and liquid I had. I gulped down some tepid chocolate milk, hardly taking a breath between long, thirsty sips. I used no water brushing my teeth, retreated into my tent, and zipped it tight.

The roads I'd been riding on were lonely and very remote, and I hadn't seen a single vehicle the whole day. I'd passed only a couple of small ranches that displayed no signs of life. But wouldn't you know it? At one in the morning, a car passed right by my camp. I woke up in full alert mode, watching the red lights retreat through the mesh of my tent. My head raised, I held as still as a lizard, listening to make sure the engine kept moving away. Soon, all was dead quiet again, but I could hear my heart loudly thumping in my throat. Had the car stopped and turned its lights off? Had they seen me? I stopped breathing. In my mind, I kept going over my escape plan, which direction I would run, and what I could quickly grab to take with me. One hand rested on my Leatherman with the knife blade open, the other on a half-full water bottle. I was ready to bolt. My breathing was shallow, and I felt like a trapped animal. Long after the car passed, I noticed I was still holding my breath and my knife. I put my head down and tried to relax. I could feel the adrenaline flowing. Somehow, I drifted back to sleep. In the morning, birds greeted the day. I was relieved to be alive, still holding onto the knife, its blade reflecting an early morning light.

As I did every morning, I sent a message to Jim via satellite: "Packing up and ready to hit the trail. All is well!" After allowing myself to heat up a cup of cocoa to complement my gourmet fried egg and tortilla breakfast, I checked out the maps on my Garmin and my iPhone. I'd carried this special egg securely wrapped in napkins and foil in my tin cup, which hung on the back of my bike. It was very precious. I heated the tortilla on the rocks, and the egg sizzled in a pan coated with olive oil. I used the same oil on my face, hands, and saddle sores. Some of the sores had scabbed over on my butt and my crotch, leaving the skin feeling rough, but new ones appeared daily, even though I was trying to constantly shift my sitting position on the saddle. My skin was dry, and my lips were cracked. I tightened the Velcro belt on both sides of my waist on my riding shorts. Warming up my toes on the rocks, which were hot from the fire, I managed to kick my cup of hot chocolate by mistake, and the whole damn thing spilled into the fire before I had a chance to catch it. Party's over! My frustrated scream drowned the morning birdsong.

"Fuuuuuck! I am so thirsty!"

A guttural cry escaped into the void as I rechecked my water supply and my maps yet again, perhaps hoping that by doing so, the distance would somehow shrink.

I was on the road around eight, before it got too hot. I needed to ride as far as possible using as little water as possible. I allowed myself the first sip at ten o'clock. To prolong the satisfaction, I held the water in my mouth for a long time before swallowing it. The temperatures crept higher, the glare from the midday sun burned my eyes, and I was down to less than one regular bike-sized bottle of precious liquid. I was afraid to look at the temperature but couldn't help myself. It was 101, and it soon topped 103. No more checking. I had forty miles to go. Every time I wiped the sweat from my eyes, burning with crusty salt, I'd see a flashing picture of my body being ripped apart by turkey vultures. I needed to take my mind off my water crisis.

"Oh, what big ears you have, señor!" I'd yell as I passed another giant cardón.

"All the better to hear you, honey," the cardón would answer.

"What big eyes you have!"

"All the better to see you."

I realized I was losing it. A laugh of desperation escaped me.

Drained of energy, dehydrated, and now feeling scared I might actually die in the heat, I sought shade under one of those giant talking cacti, which was probably over three hundred years old. As soon as I stopped, though, I was inundated by flies and bobos, these tiny pesky bugs that invaded my mouth, nostrils, ears, and eyes. I gobbled down my crackers and a can of sardines, hurrying as much as possible without eating too many bugs. Licking the can, I made sure not a drop of salty oil was left. Then a piece of a cracker got lodged in my throat. As I tried to wash it down with small sips, the water disappeared in my mouth before it even reached my parched throat. My tongue was compressed, and I could feel the indentation of my teeth in it. It was still full of tiny bumps from the cactus needles. I contemplated waiting for things to cool off, but then I'd have to ride in the dark, which I didn't want to do. I was scared. Scared that I was running out of options.

Out of the blue, a pickup truck passed by, and I saw a full case of delicious, sweet water in the bed of the truck riding away from me! I jumped up, waving and screaming frantically like a woman chased by the devil. The truck finally skidded to a stop, sending a cloud of dust into the air.

Two guys dressed in camouflage pants jumped out of the truck as The Beast and I caught up to it.

I froze. *Well, I'll either die of thirst, or these two guys will do the job!*

I was scanning them and assessing the situation.

"Hola!" They greeted me with a friendly smile, and I relaxed.

"¿Tienes un poquito agua, por favor?" I pleaded for water, full of hope. My mouth was hanging open, and I held an empty water bottle in their direction, feeling like a very desperate Oliver Twist. The guys just stared at me in bewilderment and started filling up every water bottle on my bike. Then they gave me an ice-cold bottle of lemon-flavored electrolyte drink, which I downed, hardly taking a breath. It turned out they were a support vehicle for the Baja 1000 race, which was starting in a few days. They were scoping out the roads and setting up resupply areas. I just stood there gulping warm but refreshing water. We chatted for a bit, and it turned out they were the ones who had driven by me in the middle of the night.

"There is water in the arroyo not far away, but it's not drinkable," they told me. They took pictures of me and my bike, marveling over its setup. "You are a very brave woman riding through here by yourself!"

They took off after wishing me good luck and safe travels.

Again, I'd been saved by total strangers. I stood there for a little longer, drinking more of the precious water and marveling at my fate.

When I got to the arroyo, the murky dark, slimy green water was infested with bugs and wasn't even clean enough to wash my hands. I was glad I didn't need to filter that muck, but I knew I would have done it if the guys in the truck hadn't saved me.

"We got this, Beast!" I said out loud. We both needed encouragement. My bike had become a living extension of my body, and I talked to him more often than what might seem normal. "We can ride as far as we want now that we have water."

Just like that, after several hours, we hit Mex 1 in the blazing heat. Suffocating hot air rose from the pavement. Opting to ride on the main highway, I planned to cover more ground than on the dirt road in hopes of reaching Cataviña by nightfall. I kept calculating and I thought I had between six and ten miles to go. I pumped my legs and thought of nothing. I was running on fumes.

Out of nowhere, a small truck pulled up alongside, driven by a scruffy-looking guy. He drove slowly, pushing me to the farthest edge of the road. I was teetering an inch from a steep drop-off. His rusted white truck sat low to the ground on wobbly wheels. He asked me if I needed water, signaling me to pull over. No place to do that. I didn't stop. Instead, I scanned my surroundings, pedaling faster and faster, summoning the energy created by as much as fear as anger. Ahead lay seemingly endless road entering endless hills.

"I have plenty of water!" I said, looking straight ahead and hoping he would drive away. *"Gracias, Gracias!"*

I waved him off impatiently, calling out to him in Spanish, "I am riding to Cataviña, and I am almost there!"

I took a quick glimpse at him. He gave me a toothless grin and said, *"Cataviña esta todavia muy lejos! Cincuenta kilometros!"*

Fifty kilometers? Over thirty miles? Surely, he was making that up just to make me nervous. I felt my heart race in my throat and blood pumping into my overheated temples. I pressed my lips into a tight line. Finally, a big semi-truck had to pass both of us, a reminder that trucks did pass occasionally. If I just kept riding, I'd be safe. It was getting deadly though. The Beast led me on as if riding by brail, as if he knew where to go all on his own. Neither the Garmin nor the phone helped. I couldn't take my eyes off the road to look. I had no idea how far away I was from anything. My mouth was dry, but I didn't dare to take a sip of water.

I'd always believed that there was good in everyone I met. I would finally pay the price for my naïveté. As I turned to my left again to look at the man, our eyes locked. This time, I didn't let mine drop.

"Okay, okay, amiga," he said, licking his lips with a tongue as quick as a snake's. His shifting red eyes finally let go of mine. I peddled hard. Finally, he pulled a U-turn and went back where he had come from. I didn't dare look over my shoulder for a long time, and when I did, he had disappeared into the hills behind me.

"Damn, I have to get off this main road." I said out loud, my voice shaking.

The road dipped into the arroyo, and a vulture feasted on a cow's carcass just a few feet away. As I passed, the bird cocked his red bold head, spread his giant black wings, and took off.

Not much later, at around five o'clock, the light started to make long, shifty shadows. I approached a sharp turn, and a car was pulled over just ahead of me on the right. A guy was rolling a big tire across the highway. I assumed he had a flat. Then another guy ran onto the road with a huge rock and dropped it beside the big tire. The tire and a huge rock were now lying in the middle of the lane. The two guys then jumped in the car and took off burning rubber.

"What the hell?" I said, utterly confused.

Suddenly, a car sped through the turn toward the tire and the rock. I pulled off the road in anticipation of a major accident. I frantically waved my arms and screamed, hoping the people in the oncoming car would see and hear me. I willed them to stop even though I pictured the car flying through the air in my direction.

"Oh, please stop, please stop," I pleaded.

The car slammed on the brakes and squealed to a stop just before hitting the tire and the rock. They could have been killed. I exhaled the breath I didn't know I was holding. The two men who stepped out of the car thanked me profusely for alerting them. They cleared the road, and we waved to each other, continuing our separate ways.

Mainlining adrenaline, I made it to a truck stop restaurant just before dark. Spicy beef stew and Corona revived me. The female owner pointed me to a spot behind the restaurant where I could camp. Long ago, this had served as an RV park. I was surrounded by broken trailers and a truck missing an engine. A chicken coop sat beyond the fence. Roosters with bright green feathers roamed freely. Dogs barked nearby, and my sleeping bag coaxed me into a deep sleep for most of the night, despite loud, braking trucks. It had been a long and exciting day, and I was overwhelmingly tired.

The next day at noon, I finally reached Cataviña. The toothless guy in the truck had been right: I'd completely miscalculated how far it was. I felt a pinch of guilt. Perhaps he was just trying to be helpful, but my intuition told me otherwise. I had to trust my gut feeling when I waved him away, even if I was just really worn out or if the heat and dehydration had frazzled my brain.

I passed a cheap motel on the left and instead checked into the fancy Mission Cataviña Hotel. It was packed because of the upcoming Baja 1000 race. Jim would have loved to check out all the cars and motorcycles on trailers in front of the hotel. I got the last room—a suite, large enough for the whole damn family. It was expensive, but I didn't care. I needed a break. For the first time, I sent my clothes to be laundered. When I got them back, I inhaled them like a newborn baby inhales her mother's scent. I felt reborn and rejuvenated after a bath, even though the water was just barely warm.

I went to sit by the pool and ordered a beer and chips with salsa. Life almost felt normal again. I could have used that cold swimming pool a day earlier! Lots of dudes dressed in motorcycle gear walked around, so I was not comfortable swimming in my underwear, even though I knew how invigorating jumping into cold water would feel. When I logged onto the hotel Wi-Fi, a text message from my dear friend Marilyn, who has been like a mother to me since college, popped up: "My daughter has just been diagnosed with breast cancer. You should call her if you can."

I immediately dialed my friend's daughter, Stephanie, in San Francisco, and we talked for a long time. I felt her pain and fear of the unknown, as I thought back to that initial shock of the doctor's confirming my diagnosis. I replayed the sound of the tiny bird slamming against my glass door—that feeling of your lungs filling with ice water. She was still waiting for surgery to remove the tumor and the biopsy results so they could decide on the course of treatment.

"I am just going to have both of my breasts removed," she said. "I want to be safe."

I remembered that sense of urgency. I counseled her to take her time making big decisions. It's difficult to wait, but I told her she'd know much more after the test results came.

"The waiting is dreadful," I said. "All that uncertainty; thinking your life is over. But you have the best doctors and hospitals around you. You are in good hands."

Deciding what to do with my breasts was one of the most painful aspects of my diagnosis. Yes, I wanted to do everything possible to survive, but I was quite attached to my breasts as well. I worried about how Jim would feel if they were gone. Would he still be attracted to me? Would he still love me? My boobs were on the smaller side, but despite my age and breastfeeding three kids, they still looked perky, the breasts of an athlete. Hearing from Jim that it didn't matter to him whether I had one, two, one and a half, or no breasts made all the difference to me on the first meeting with our surgeon. I opted to not have reconstructive surgery. At that time, I had too many other things on my plate.

I felt sad for Stephanie. I knew she faced difficult times, and nothing I said would change that. She had to get through it. Luckily, she had a great support network of family and friends, which is crucial. What made me feel a bit better was that my trip seemed to inspire her. She saw that she would get through it and would be able to go back to doing the things she loved.

I made no plans for the rest of my journey. The route before me was long and remote. There was a two-, perhaps a three-day section along the Pacific coast without water resupply for a hundred miles. I couldn't decide if I should ride it or skip it. I was nervous but confident that the way forward would present itself. For now, I needed to rest and lift my dampened spirits. I needed to revive my tired body. I needed to be good to myself.

—TWENTY-THREE—
Divine Intervention

*The vicissitudes of the road have a wonderful talent
for bringing out the fine flavor of character.*
—Gertrude Bell, nineteenth-century traveler

Life can be reduced to simple things that give us pleasure. I was living one of those magical moments. I was alone in the desert, a tiny speck of utter insignificance in our grand universe, reclining under stars and constellations I wished I could name. A bat flew over my head as the fire died down. I sipped a cup of miso soup. I saw the Big Dipper and the Little Dipper and traced the sky from Polaris to the brightest star, Sirius, the big dog of them all. Luminous balls of gas, thousands of light-years away. The life cycle of a star spans billions of years, so what am I doing here? What do I represent?

I've sworn I would never allow myself to be hurt again. I've asked for mercy not to be tested anymore. So, there I was, searching for meaning, looking to belong. I felt something shift deep inside. I found consolation in the sky and felt the grandeur of the universe, the stars winking at me like they were saying, *You got this, girl! Keep on moving forward. You matter. You do have a spirit, which belongs to the greater universe!*

Suddenly, a shooting star flashed across the sky.

I didn't make a wish. I didn't need to.

I was living my dream right then and there. I was so grateful that I was still alive at that very moment in space and time. I was glad I hadn't quit riding. I would have missed so many beautiful and powerful moments like the one I was experiencing. I felt that things were really coming together. I felt immense pride in what I was achieving. I was tired but surprisingly not exhausted from the day's seventy-mile ride. My body was strong and getting stronger by the day. Most importantly, my confidence in myself and in greater humanity was returning. I was starting to better understand why the urge to make this pilgrimage was so strong, but this was coming to me intuitively, emotionally, not in a way I could explain in words.

My campsite was tucked under spectacularly shaped granite boulders. The one above my tent looked like Pride Rock from Disney's *Lion King.*

I donned my bike gloves and began carefully gathering firewood. I was in scorpion country, and they love to hang out in rotting branches. As I threw wood onto the fire, they scurried out of the burning wood into the desert night.

Autumn had arrived, even here in the desert. With the time change, it was getting dark early. I retreated to my tent at seven o'clock to get away from mosquitoes, and the night was peaceful. At some point, I realized even the crickets had quieted down. A bat diving for mosquitoes flew so close over the tent that I could hear the *whoosh* of the air on the silky-thin fabric. Coyotes yelped in the near distance. The night belonged to them, but it belonged to me as well. I was grateful to all the creatures around me that were sharing their home. I heard the occasional hoot of an owl, and I felt safe and warm in my cocoon.

By eight the next morning, I was riding toward Bahía de Los Ángeles. The road stretched before me, lined by cirios. My mood paralleled the aura of my surroundings, and I hollered at the top of my lungs. No one but The Beast heard me.

Energy released from every pore of my body. It was pure ecstasy, pure joy. I'd found the happiness I'd been seeking, if only for a fleeting moment, and I knew that if I didn't pay attention, it would vanish. Happiness is not perpetual and long lasting. Happiness is a precise moment we create. I alone created that happiness on a desolate stretch of road leading me to the Sea of Cortez.

At noon, after only thirty-four and a half miles, The Beast and I reached the Sea of Cortez in the Bay of Los Ángeles. I headed north about a mile out of town to a campground. It was a pleasant place and, as I didn't have any other options, I set up camp. But I'd made a mistake not buying any food or water in town. I thought there'd be a restaurant, or a little convenience store at the campground, but only one other trailer was parked there.

Inside were Kent and Lilian, a very nice couple who by utter coincidence were traveling from British Columbia to La Ventana, my second home. All of a sudden, the campground took on the rosy hue of familiar friends. They gave me a ride to town to get supplies and invited me over to a lovely dinner. Lilian was originally from Sweden and, boy, was it ever so nice to sit at a table in a spotless trailer, eat good food, drink wine, and have a compelling and intelligent conversation. We found an instant connection, and we had much in common, and even their small shih tzu dog, Elmo, slowly got used to me.

Afterward, the gentle sound of waves lulled me to sleep. The air was calm, and bright stars speckled a moonless sky. Dawn arrived at five in the morning. I caught that glorious moment, that time just before sunrise. The sky turned crimson, slowly changing from blood red to softer pinks. I lingered in my sleeping bag with the tent doors unzipped and framing the bay. Gulls squawked, and brown pelicans plunged into the sea for their breakfast. What a show!

And then—just to spoil the perfect morning—my stove wouldn't work. Again. I really wanted to enjoy a hot cup of coffee with the sunrise.

"You piece of shit!" I scolded the damned thing, then started taking it apart piece by piece and managed to get it working. By the time I was finished, I'd lost the desire to get on the road.

My tent and the riding shorts I'd washed the night before were saturated with dew. A heavy mist enshrouded the bay during the night. My decision to stay came quickly, and I was content with it. Kent and Lilian picked me up with their truck, and we spent a pleasant day on Gringa beach and estuary, swimming and snorkeling and watching gulls fight for fish. Meanwhile, a stately and elegant blue heron, ever so watchful, looked at its own reflection in waters slightly rippled by an easterly breeze. Lilian served us peanut butter sandwiches, cold water, and watermelon for lunch. I felt like a kid adopted by the kindest of foster parents.

Riding my bike every day and constantly moving forward, I realized I'd forgotten how to be still. My body and mind were grateful. When we returned to the campground, we planned to take a quick shower before heading to town for supper. I got to my tent and had to fix some stakes that pulled out. I wondered how that happened? I crawled into the tent to get my clothes and a towel to go take a shower and to my horror, noticed big slashes and holes in the mesh wall! It looked like curiosity got the better of Tuna, a very friendly four-month-old puppy who roamed around freely and belonged to the campground owners. I was not happy at all! I wondered if I should say anything. What would I do for a tent? This was my home and sanctuary in a land infested with bugs and mosquitoes. Luckily, I had a sewing kit, so I put on my broken reading glasses and quickly got to work to sewing the gaps just before dark. There was no time to take a shower before we headed to town for dinner. Normally, that wouldn't faze me, but I so craved the luxury!

In the morning, I was ready for an early start at six. My damn stove was on strike yet again. I gave up on it and decided to just cook on a fire whenever I could. While walking to the bathroom, I saw another van parked a few sites down from me. The guys asked me if I needed anything, and I said, "Yeah, a cup of coffee would be nice." One of the men, whose name was Simon, kindly obliged while I was explaining my stove failure. Turns out he was the head of an outdoor program at a university and knew quite a few things about camp stoves.

He took mine apart, explaining everything about each piece as he went. Then he put it back together again. It worked for a bit, then died. We repeated the cleaning process several times, and then he taught me how to pull the cable out to clean CO_2 debris clogging the flow of the fuel. I felt I was now intimately connected with each little piece of the finicky device, and I had passed a crash course, Stove Maintenance 101.

Two hours later, I was finally on the road. It was a late start, but I was grateful for all the new information. I hoped it meant the stove and I would be starting a new relationship.

Bumping along, the washboard took me south from Bahía de Los Ángeles on a gentle climb through a beautiful Cardonales, a forest of giant cardón cacti. Hundreds of turkey vultures perched on the tips of the arms of these magnificent plants, some of which reached as high as sixty feet. The vultures stood guard as I rode by, motionless, with their large black wings spread wide and with their backs to the sun. I suspected they were following me, waiting for their opportunity to feast upon my body.

The small plastic Garmin computer that was strapped to my mountain bike handlebar like a watch read 106 degrees. That was all I could think about. I had to cover forty-six miles to my next stop in San Rafael Bay. There would be no supplies there, so I also had to ration my water, and that is not an easy thing to do when sweat is gushing out of every pore. I pushed The Beast up yet another impossibly steep hill to ride over the endless, rough, bumpy road. All I wanted to do was drink. As dehydration pushed me nearly into delirium, I pictured a water hose attached straight to my vein, while images of hospital gowns and chemo treatments haunted me. Water, water, water!

Palo verde trees lined the road through lush desert, but they didn't provide a lick of shade. At the halfway point, I finally found a tree big enough to hide from the sun, cool down, and have a snack of rice pudding and water. Green mold had grown around the edges of the pudding, but minor details like that didn't matter. To my road-weary body, it tasted delicious. A gentle breeze cooled the air just enough that it would have been pleasant, if not for buzzing flies, mosquitoes, and bobos. It was impossible to avoid swallowing them along with the food I shoved in my mouth. I had to keep moving.

The sun dipped below the horizon before I reached San Rafael Bay. Silhouettes of the mountains etched themselves into the blood-orange skyline. I stopped to try to take a photo, but mosquitoes swarmed me, so I kept moving. The sound of a motorcycle sent me scrambling off the dirt road behind a giant cardón, its thick trunk and multiple branches offering safe shelter. I quickly turned off my headlamp, holding my breath. Three dirt bike riders passed by and continued in the opposite direction. A frightened jackrabbit scurried between my feet and brushed against my bare skin with his large ears. I let out a muffled scream, my hands gripping the handlebar tightly, my heart thumping in my chest. I waited until the dirt bikers' red lights disappeared before I got back on the road, which finally dropped me down to the water's edge in darkness. I passed a fishing shack of a few old plywood boards, some cardboard pieces in between to fill the gaps, and a rusted tin roof.

"Buenas noches," I greeted the fisherman sitting in front of his shelter, smoking and staring into the darkness. All I saw at first was the red glow of his cigarette. I realized I had startled him. Before he was even able to reply, a soldier in full attire, including a machine gun strapped across his chest, appeared from a thicket. In the beam of my headlight, he towered over me like a demon. I could feel his soured cigarette breath on my face, and somehow, I managed to hold on to the bike and not fall over.

"Jeez!" I gasped, sucking the air out of my toes. I smiled, faking confidence. I greeted him in a friendly way as my eyes took a quick look at the nametag on his left chest. "Ma . . . nez" was all I could see. He noticed I was trying to read his nametag.

"Sargento Martinez," he said, introducing himself sharply. *"¿Qué Haces aquí?"* "What are you doing here?"

I tried to decipher the tone of his voice.

"Hola! Donde puedo acampar, Sargento Martinez?" Hi! Where can I camp, Sergeant Martinez?

As I tried to catch my breath, those words were the first thing that came to my mind, and I managed to ask him in as friendliest voice I could muster.

He pointed me down to the crescent-shaped, white sandy beach, and with a sweeping motion of his hand, exclaimed, *"Es todo tuyo!"* It's all yours.

Then he looped his thumbs around his gun belt and looked at the bay with admiration as if he owned the whole place himself. I glanced at the profile of his large head. He had a big confidant smile. I relaxed and felt safer having soldiers around, not just a lone fisherman.

This was all mine! The whole eerily empty, beautiful, and lonely bay.

It was barely seven o'clock, but I was engulfed in the darkness, the sky littered with stars. Yes, it was all mine! This whole trip I'd decided to embark on alone. After fifty-four years, I felt I was alone for the first time in my life. This was me, here and now! My husband was not standing next to me to protect me. None of my kids were there needing my protection. I was alone with this fully loaded heavy bike I pushed every day. Alone with cracked lips, windblown and unwashed hair sticking in all directions, sweat and dust caked on skin as dry as parchment. Alone in the unrelentingly hot days and bone-chilling nights. I was also alone with constant lack of water and food when I rode endless miles on remote dirt roads, not knowing where I'd find supplies or a place to set up the tent. I lived alone with the fear of the unknown, the unplanned, the unrecognizable, and the unpredictable which were shaping every moment of my journey. I was alone in the company of the mosquitoes, snakes, and scorpions. And I was alone with the fear of a little bunny running between my feet, most likely much more scared than I.

I pushed The Beast through soft sand and found a spot in the shelter of a panga, a typical Mexican fishing boat. This one had no engine, so I knew the fisherman would not be taking it out early. I quickly set up the tent, and then struggled with my ever-failing stove in hopes of heating some soup. I gave up after several attempts, cursing loudly. When I heard chuckles up on the hill, I realized I was being watched. The tent, as always, was a sanctuary I could crawl into and hide, not just from mosquitoes, but also from the rest of the world. I could surround myself with the flimsy fabric and have the illusion that I was protected from the hostile environment on the other side of the mesh. But hostility was only a product of my own mind.

My thoughts followed me everywhere. Listening to the waves gently lapping onto the sandy beach just feet away, I drifted off to sleep chewing on a cold, dry tortilla and a slimy dark banana. The smell of it made me nauseous, yet I was too hungry not to eat it. At three in the morning, when sleep eluded me again, my thoughts grew darker, and fear oozed into my aching muscles. The inflamed femoral nerve of my damaged right leg felt as if hot lava were flowing through it. That screaming pain woke me. Like every goddamn night! My quad muscle at the front of my thigh was as hard as a rock and pulsing in spasmodic pain. I lay down on my back moaning, breathing deep, slow breaths until the cramp finally loosened its grip. I counted the waves; I counted the stars; I counted the bunnies with long ears darting across the desert; I counted the sand kernels in my sleeping bag; I counted my breaths. Nothing worked. I was relieved when morning gray light finally started to seep in. I'd made it through yet another mostly sleepless night.

By the time the sun rose, my jumbled thoughts had washed into the sea. Now that I was an expert, I took my stove apart and finally had the soup I'd mixed the night before. The sergeant came back for a visit with two soldiers, young boys the age of my son. They admired my bike. They also were interested in my Garmin navigation and Mini InReach satellite devices. They took photos of both and discussed possibilities for the army to purchase them, so they asked me how much they cost. It made me wonder though, if something were to happen to me and I had to use the SOS feature on my satellite device, would these be the guys who would come rescue me? Would they have a way to find my coordinates? They were not familiar with the unit, and when I tried to explain to the sergeant how the SOS feature worked, he didn't seem to have a clue who would contact them if the need arose. I realized it's best not to test my fate. I had to remain self-reliant. I must not get hurt. It's just as simple as that. The guys wanted to take photos of The Beast and me.

"*Buena suerte, loca!*"

They wished me, this crazy woman from far, far away, a safe trip.

I packed slowly, went for a refreshing dip in the ocean, aware the whole time the soldiers were watching from the hill, and reluctantly got back on the bike. I had a short day ahead, or so I thought. It was only twenty-five miles over a pass to Rancho Escondido, which had food, beer, and rooms for rent. Supposedly. I pictured myself sitting in the shade, eating tacos, and enjoying a cold beer. In my mind, it was always a bottle of Corona with a lime wedged perfectly balanced on top, a sandy beach, a sun umbrella, and turquoise ocean waters in the background. That got me moving. The power of commercials! I pedaled inland, watching the temperature steadily rise.

There is an intricate balance between life and death in the desert. Fragility and ruggedness walk hand in hand. Water is the crucial source of life, and nowhere was that more apparent than in arid Southern Baja. Recent rains painted the desert in vivid greens, bright reds, eye-blinding yellows, and soft purples. I had yet to identify the source of the opulent sweet smells, but I suppose that didn't really matter. If I had been passing through in a closed air-conditioned car, I wouldn't have smelled anything. Riding my mountain bike out there at my own pace, I felt the caress of the sweet air on my sweaty body.

After all the miles, my mind often went blank, which led to me pedaling as if I were on autopilot. The Beast and I were in tune with each other. On easier stretches of the trails, I could surrender to the unconscious mind and sink into a thoughtless world. It often felt as if I were in a deep state of meditation, and everything around me stopped existing. Often, several hours passed without me noticing. On a gentle downslope, I enjoyed the effortless movement, and without warning, as I was not paying attention, a giant rattlesnake appeared, stretched from one side of the trail to the other, blocking my path. Too late to stop or change course, I ran over the poor unsuspecting creature. It coiled up quickly, ready to strike, and instinctively I lifted my feet way up into the air, nearly losing balance. Loaded on adrenaline, I sped away from it as fast as I could.

"Shit, shit, shit!" I screamed out loud, riding as if a fire-breathing dragon were chasing me. "Sorry, sorry, sorry!" I kept screaming, apologizing to the snake as thick as my arm. I turned around just to catch the snake slithering off the gravel road, disappearing among the cholla cacti. I was glad I didn't hurt it. I was the intruder in her peaceful world. I had rudely interrupted her midmorning lounging in the sun.

After that, I was a lot more alert. A pleasant meandering road started climbing and brought me over the pass to a granite boulder plateau. It was densely populated by a variety of cacti, trees, and blooming flowers. I wished I had room to carry a book so I could identify them all. I stopped for water as the temperature rose to over a hundred degrees again. I was not saving water. I only had about five miles to go. I took my time. I indulged my senses by listening to a variety of birdsong. I closed my eyes, and when I opened them, a red fox was trotting along the road just a few feet away. As soon as it sensed me, it turned around, ears pointing straight up, and stared at me for a long moment. We were checking each other out. I wanted it to stay, but it hurried into the forest of the high desert. I inhaled deeply and climbed back on The Beast. I could hear that cold Corona calling.

I came to an intersection with signs pointing to Rancho Escondido. In English, it would be called Hidden Ranch. When I followed the sign, my Garmin started beeping, telling me I was off course. I kept turning around and then got back on track on a smaller, more rugged road through the thick growth. *This must be the road to the ranch*, I thought. I could already see myself sitting at the table, eating good food and drinking cold beer, chatting with rancheros. But then, I was suddenly back on the main road. It looked like I'd taken a shortcut. I must be almost there! The road was soft and sandy, going uphill, so I was making painfully slow progress. My spirits dampened, as I thought I'd be there already. Something was rotten in the land of Baja. I sent Jim a message via satellite: "Sweetheart, can you tell on the map if I've passed the ranch?"

Luckily, he was home, and he confirmed my suspicions after he consulted the maps. He texted back: "You passed the ranch by a couple of miles,

Shit. Not what I wanted to hear!

I turned around and slogged back through the soft sand; however, now I was going downhill, which helped.

I was just about there when a car came toward me. I flagged it down to confirm that I was heading in the right direction to Rancho Escondido. The driver said, "Yes, but there is no one there. The ranch is closed. The owners went to Ensenada."

This was not good news. I was down to one bottle of water and a can of tuna. I'd eaten only soup and some nuts along the way. I'd been counting on food and water at the ranch. The next place was eighteen and a half miles up the hill, over a pass on a road covered in deep sand. It was three o'clock, which meant I had only two hours of light left. There was no way I could make that. He offered me a ride to Rancho Piedra Blanco, which I gladly accepted.

"*¿Cerveza?*" Beer? He offered.

"*Muchísimos gracias!*" Thank you so much! Hell yeah, tepid beer and a ride in the car? I'll take it!

Angel lived on a ranch in San Franciscito with his mother. He was traveling to Guerrero Negro to visit his father and to get supplies for the ranch. The back of his car was packed full, and he had a large barrel for fuel, which took up much of the space. Somehow, we made enough room to stuff The Beast into the back of his SUV after I removed the front wheel. Some things fell off the bike as we forcefully shoved it in. I didn't care. I'd deal with it later.

Call it divine intervention. I'll just say I got my ass saved again by an angel. At Piedra Blanca ranch, I bought Angel a case of beer, and the lady of the ranch got a ride with him to Guerrero Negro just after she fixed me a plate of four small burritos. The traditional burritos were just a tortilla wrapped around beans or shredded beef called *machaca*. They prepared their machaca the traditional way by drying seasoned beef in the sun and shredding it. It lasts a long time without needing refrigeration.

The ranchers in the area live miles apart, but they all know each other, mostly through family connections, and are interdependent. They communicate via CB radio.

However, even in those remote areas, localism was slowly disappearing and, with it, its unique character. I passed and stayed in places where very modest homes had no running water, trash was littered everywhere, yet kids were running around with iPhones and iPads.

I enjoyed a cold beer at my little casita, some simple food, a hot shower, and a bed. Life was good again! As I lay in bed that night, I wondered how I'd managed to get lost. I read trail directions for that section several times while I was on a break in Bahía de Los Ángeles. Chemo had fried my brain, and my memory was awful. As I reread the directions, it all came back to me. The shortcut I took bypassed the ranch. Damn it! I'd been frustrated and scared. I could not rely on my memory alone. I had to check maps and notes more carefully. I could not make a mistake. I might not get another chance. So many had died before me. So many I'd known in my life or read about, missed that second chance. I didn't come here to die. I came here to live. People often think that climbers, extreme skiers, explorers of the dangerous and unknown worlds all have a death wish. But I know it is quite the opposite. They have a desire to live a more meaningful life by living closer to the edge, where they can see life more clearly.

—TWENTY-FOUR—
Another Nightmare

Sleep, delicious and profound, the very counterfeit of death.
—Homer, *The Odyssey*

Alejandro was a slight man. He had been living on a ranch for more than forty years. Most of his teeth were gone, which made him look older than he probably was and hard to understand. The language spoken by the local mountain people was challenging to comprehend regardless. They ate half their words. Much of the conversation depended on picking up on body language, intuition, and lots of nodding with a blank expression, pretending I knew what they were saying. He filled my bottles with sweet water that came from a well six hundred feet deep. The ranch also had solar and wind power.

Everything was immaculate and clean and raked. It was a most pleasant place, surrounded by massive white granite boulders and cardón. The cabins were clean and straightforward. The deep well provided the ranch with plenty of water. The family who lived on the ranch was entirely self-sufficient. They had to be to survive that far away from any city. Only rarely, to get supplies or for other exceptions, did they descend into the town of Guerrero Negro, which was several hours away by car.

Alejandro leaned the rake against the railing and invited me to sit on his veranda. He motioned me toward a wooden chair next to a long table, which had undoubtedly hosted many a family gathering. The screen door creaked and slammed behind him when he went into the kitchen. He returned with two glasses of fresh limeade, made from the bright green limes that grew on the tree behind the house, and sat in his rocking chair.

"I am content up here," he said, without my prompting him. "I have everything I need. My family, my work, my land. You gringos, you are always going somewhere. Don't you have a family?"

He reached up with his calloused hand and adjusted his white cowboy hat. His eyes, the color of chocolate, scanned the perimeter. Alejandro's young and handsome son, or more likely a grandson, tended cattle in the corral.

"I never go to the city," he said calmly. "The young ones sometimes do, but my heart and soul are here."

It occurred to me that Alejandro just told me the secret of life that I'd been searching for.

The strange thing is that I didn't even know I had been looking for it.

By leading a hardworking yet simple life at home, he was surrounded by beautiful, harsh nature and, most importantly, his family. That is what made him happy. That was all he needed. Was that all I needed? Truly? Did I ride all these endless miles to find Alejandro to tell me this? Just like Emerson walked a hundred miles through a snowstorm for one good conversation, I realized I had to ride more than a thousand miles to hear Alejandro tell me he was content in his *home*.

I understood in that instant that home was not a physical space. I'd left a loving, safe, and stable home in Slovenia. I will always think of that as my primary home. It's where I was born, where my parents and family live. Then I built my first home with my first husband. It didn't last, but I can still hear the children's laughter echoing through each room. I'd lost the home I rebuilt for my kids and myself after the divorce to the banks. Now I was so far away from the one I created with Jim, yet I still had him, my children, and the rest of my family constantly with me as I traveled through these remote, harsh, yet beautiful places.

Home is a state of mind.

Home is where you feel safe and loved, where it smells of fresh-baked bread, family and friends gather around the table, and the fireplace keeps everyone warm. They fight about politics, yet still hug each other when bellies are full, the last bottle of wine is empty, and the dirty dishes are stacked in the sink.

I wanted to chat more with Alejandro, spend a day with him, explore the area. I wanted to visit the life-sized rock paintings he told me were nearby and to meet the rest of his family. I questioned why I didn't stay longer in some of these beautiful places. But I was in a hurry, in part, because I wanted to meet up with Jim. Even though I thought I would return someday, deep down, I knew I never would. Just like Alejandro said, "You gringos are always going somewhere."

I felt a new lightness as I rode toward El Arco. Everything looked beautiful. Alejandro had pointed out the truth with one simple sentence. But I realized it was something I already knew. It had been there my whole life.

I pulled to the side of the road and sat in the shade of a lonely tree. I snacked on nuts and realized I'd lost yet another water bottle. Surprisingly I was not worried about it. Somehow nothing seemed like a problem. I knew that someone would come by sooner or later, offer help, and save me.

In El Arco, I decided to ride southwest toward Mex 1 to avoid a ten-mile sandy stretch I'd been warned about by an experienced dirt biker. He had been loud and confident, so I took him at his word.

When I finally reached Mex 1, there was no place to resupply. After the forty-three miles I'd already ridden, I had thirty miles on a road without any shoulder to reach the agricultural town of Vizcaíno. I rode as close to the edge of the highway as possible, but I was incredibly nervous and uncomfortable because it dropped off at least two feet. My heavy bike swayed every time a truck passed.

It sucked! I shouldn't have listened to the advice to avoid the sandy road. I might have pushed the bike, but it would have been much safer. After I'd ridden several unsafe miles, a bright red pickup stopped, and a guy offered me a ride.

"*Peligroso, peligroso!*" he shouted out of his window, pointing at my bike and the back of his truck. "Come, come!"

He'd stopped in the middle of the lane, so a big semi-truck had to pass by crossing into the oncoming lane. I had to decide on the spot. I accepted the offer as it was getting late, the light was fading, and he felt genuine. Besides, camping on the side of the road was out of the question. Still, I was aware of how dumb it was to accept a ride on a Mexican highway from a stranger driving a fancy red pickup.

Roberto introduced himself while we were quickly loading the bike on the back of his pickup. He chatted excitedly, in a nonthreatening manner, but the whole time he talked, I was going over my escape plan and reasoning with myself.

Don't worry. He wouldn't have stopped if he didn't want to help you! He's a good guy! He's a family man. But I also thought to myself, *These might be your famous last words!* I sat in the passenger seat on my hands and listened to Roberto's rambling. I was literally looking out the window for a place to jump out of a moving vehicle. I visualized jumping, tucking and rolling once I hit the ground, hoping I wouldn't land on a cactus.

It was hard to understand Roberto's very rapid Spanish, but I learned that he was the youngest of eleven kids in the family and an avid dirt bike rider. Roberto was familiar with all the back roads around the area and confirmed that the dirt road I was supposed to ride on was indeed very sandy and barely passable. While he was driving, he was showing me photos of his family vacation to Disneyland on his iPhone. I looked at the pictures quickly, pleading with him to keep his eyes on the road. We arrived at Vizcaíno in no time. Roberto treated me to a pizza when we arrived at his place, proudly named "Roberto's Pizza." I bought him and his cousins who worked at the pizza restaurant a case of beer. I was happy to be safe, but my legs were still shaky. In my mind, I scolded myself for doubting this good man who helped me and got me off the busy and dangerous road. Fear is so ingrained. I really want to believe in the good of people.

I asked about the cheapest motel in town and he pointed me to one on a narrow side street. A motel for fifteen dollars is as cheap as it gets, but you get what you pay for. A real shower, however, after a whole day riding on dusty roads in the heat, was heaven. It didn't matter how fancy a faucet hot water flowed from. I was grateful. I watched the movie *The Perfect Storm* in Spanish. I always was grateful for a dose of George Clooney delivered in any language. Besides, I even picked up a new word or two. The sheets smelled of old cigarette smoke, but the most important thing was that I was safe.

I had fallen victim to anticipation. Any trip is a state of mind. I might anticipate that a day will not be long or difficult, but then it will become impossibly long and challenging. Seldom does it work the other way around. Traveling by bike is mentally strenuous, and of course, a million times slower than by car. You feel every little hill that is unnoticeable when you drive. The ride toward San Ignacio was one of those days. After leaving Vizcaíno, for some reason, my Garmin froze, I missed the turnoff to the dirt road. Instead of turning around and backtracking, I convinced myself it would save me many miles, that it would shorten my trip and make for an easy day. I ended up riding Mex 1 for a good part of the way. It did cut off about ten miles, but it played a dirty trick on my mind. I thought it would have gone by much faster. I couldn't wait for the ride on the main road to be over. I didn't like the trucks and cars whizzing by.

Just shy of San Ignacio I went through a standard military inspection. The soldiers asked regular questions: "Where are you from? Where are you going?"

Finally, they pointed to a camper behind me and asked me if I was with them.

"*No, viaje sola.*" No, I am traveling alone.

"*¿Sola!?*" Alone?

The soldiers chuckled.

I rode to Casa de Ciclista in the oasis of San Ignacio, which, of course, catered to cyclists. I'd heard from a truck driver in Santo Tomas about this French couple in their early seventies riding down Mex 1 ahead of me. We finally crossed paths as we were setting up our tents for the night. I never learned their names. They were farmers in their own country and were traveling through the US from Alaska via the Great Divide, all the way to Ushuaia at the southern end of Argentina. They anticipated arriving by Christmas the following year. They planned to stay on some farm cooperatives in Mexico, Cuba, Bolivia, and Columbia. Oh, I thought, I would love to ride all the way to Ushuaia with them!

We all agreed that Mexico was safer than any US city, and the people we'd met had been genuine and kind.

"I feel guilty doubting Roberto yesterday." I said to the man, who was very wiry and thin, with thinning, long gray hair.

"I think it's normal to feel that way," he said. "You're a woman, traveling alone. We are two people, traveling together. It's different. You should be careful. You should stay vigilant."

I chatted with the man while his wife was taking a shower. Unfortunately, we were not able to ride together as they were traveling on the main road, and I continued following dirt roads along the Pacific before I headed back into the mountains. I walked to the center of town in search of a restaurant. By the time I returned, they were asleep in their tent, and they left before I rose. I felt bad I never said goodbye or exchanged contact information. I thought of them often as I peddled and hoped they were safe on their journey.

San Ignacio is a charming, date palm oasis with a grand eighteenth-century mission. The site of the mission was known to local Indians as Kadakaaman, which in Cochimí language means "stream of reeds." Like many other parts of Baja as well as the rest of Latin America, the indigenous population had been wiped out by epidemic disease or absorbed into the mixed race of mestizo families, which took over the way of life.

I had a fish and rice dinner in the plaza while kids ran in the park, and pleasant Mexican music wafted from the restaurant. The first sliver of the moon traveled over the mission. The scene was romantic, even idyllic, but it was getting lonely eating alone. It would have been nice to share a pleasant evening with someone other than mosquitoes.

The next morning, the roosters and chickens started in early, and at six thirty, church bells confirmed the new day. I felt I'd been transported to Slovenia, where I woke to church bells every morning. On that Sunday, I had a quiet breakfast in the plaza accompanied by

Esnicker, an adorable, silver pit bull. He kept placing his large face in my lap and looking up at me pleadingly for food scraps.

My stay at San Ignacio was complete. Even the pit bull was friendly. I felt reasonably rested and planned a ride of about thirty miles to Laguna San Ignacio that I hoped would be easy. I knew I should have had no expectations, but I was trying to plan shorter days when possible. It was becoming clear that I needed to pace myself. The road toward Laguna was paved and quiet. I stopped at a store in San Zacarias to get water and food. People dressed in their Sunday finery lined up in front of the store. It was a local election day. I spoke with a few people on the street about the crazy politics of their northern neighbor country. I signed my name into the Baja Divide book at the store and wrote in my Slovenian nationality. The man at the counter knew precisely that Slovenia was next to Croatia, Italy and Austria, and he knew the history of Yugoslavia and its leader, Tito.

Every creature was a welcome sight on the lonely road, so I delighted in the company of a citrus-colored butterfly that rode for a moment on top of my bike pack. The thermal winds blowing from the cool Pacific into the desert, which was quickly warming, were not much of a favor. Every so often, when I crested a hump in the road, Laguna appeared a bit closer. The straight road disappeared on the horizon in the shimmering heat of midday.

I reached Laguna just past noon. It was sweltering and not a tree in sight to offer shade. I was hoping to see a whale, but at one of the fishing shacks, the local man informed me that whales had not yet arrived. Therefore, the place was deserted. I saw a few plywood shacks and a tiny store that sold mainly sodas and beer. No place to stay there, so I continued. I rode through another community, a rather large one with a school and lots of houses, mostly built from a mishmash of plywood and tin, yet painted in vivid colors. There was also a store, but it was closed on Sundays.

"Just my luck," I muttered to myself as I got off the bike.

A woman inside noticed me and opened the store. I bought a beer, a small chunk of cheese, an avocado, an apple, and a lime, all for a bit over a dollar. The shopkeepers were a lovely family who had just returned from church service. A young boy named Alejandro admired The Beast. They all wanted to know how much the bike cost, and as usual, I dodged the question. I saddled the bike and continued, as there was no place to stay, and I looked forward to the solitude of the wide-open spaces ahead.

I rode fifty feet below sea level through hostile salt flats devoid of vegetation and birds. The air was rich, smelling of salt, sand, and sea. Butter-colored sunlight deepened as the sun traveled lower on the horizon, promising a beautiful sunset. I was on the lookout for a place to camp. No trees, no hills, not even a bump. Then I spotted it in the distance. A solitary miniature Banyan tree, my oasis for the night. I slogged through soft sand away from the road and set up my tent. Not exactly hidden, but I thought I was far enough away from the sand-packed road. It was too windy to start a fire, and I didn't really want to attract attention. The few cars that passed on the firm sand of the salt flats were not far away.

I told myself they were probably just fishermen traveling home to one of the ejidos, trying to dismiss the discomfort of being so exposed. The sunset was beautiful, and after the ocean absorbed the last of the light, I crawled into the tent, lay down on my pad, and munched on a cold tortilla, fresh cheese, and avocado with lime. The beer I'd bought a few hours ago was not exactly cold but tasted excellent, nonetheless. Turning to lie on my back, I managed to spill it inside the tent, so all my stuff was swimming in beer. Great! I wiped it with a towel as best I could but was too tired to worry about it. The flysheet flapping in the wind did not keep me awake.

I had a nightmare about my daughter Jana ending up in my small tent with me, and in a panic, she woke me up saying someone was walking around outside the tent. I startled myself awake. My mind started racing. I knew I was awake as I was alone. My hand rested on my knife with its sharp double-edged blade open, but the pepper spray was on the bike outside. Again! What good was any of that going to do me anyway? All was quiet but for a soft flapping of the paper-thin walls of my tent, providing only an illusion of protection. I held my breath, listening, unable to move. My heart pulsed in my throat; every fiber of every muscle in my exhausted body was strung as tight as a violin string on the brink of snapping. I tried to recall my surroundings, my memory frozen by fear.

I was hours away from any village or even a lonesome fishing hut. If I had to run, which way would I go? Had I woken up because some-one was walking around the tent, or was it just in my dream? I heard faint sounds nearby. Slowly unzipping the tent, I peeked out. I saw nothing. Then a twig snapped, and my head jerked in the direction of the sound. My eyes straining in the darkness were following the crunching sounds. A cow emerged from the low brush, then another and another. I dropped my head into my hands in relief and then went outside to pee. The simple act of looking at the sky calmed me down.

The moon was just reaching the edge of the sky, which spanned the entire horizon, and was littered with blinking bright stars. Just breathing, I sat outside, taking in the quiet surroundings. The silence was deafening. It spilled to the outer edges of the space, which was flat as the reflection of the unrefined soul. I was deeply aware that I was all alone. It was eerie and beautiful at the same time. I was lucky to spot a couple of shooting stars. The wind died down. I gathered a handful of dried twigs from a low brush to build a tiny fire in a hole in the sand. I held the last light of the moon in the palms of my hands. The soft, milky light seeped through my fingers and then disappeared. I sat with my fire and thoughts of my children. The twigs were now just glowing embers, so I buried them with the sand, and after I'd calmed down enough, I crawled back into the tent.

Soon, my breathing coincided with the slow rhythm of the tent flapping in the gentle breeze: *caflap, caflap, caflap.* For some unknown reason, the image of Jana, my second baby, came back, haunting my every thought. Why had she visited me in my dream? She is sensitive, but by no means fragile. She is an old soul and often a protecting mother of us all.

Still, I always want to protect her.

When I was in third grade, I was rushed to the hospital by ambulance in the middle of the night with a burst appendix. Nearly dying, I suffered kidney complications afterward and needed kidney surgery a few months later. After several days in the ICU, I was begging the doctor to get me out of there into a regular room. Right across from my bed, there was a two-year-old child with severe hydrocephalus. I was terrified of him, especially at night. Visions of his tiny body and his huge head gave me nightmares for years.

Those same nightmares followed me into my pregnancy with Jana. An ultrasound at eighteen weeks showed enlarged ventricles on the baby's brain. That was a sign of possible hydrocephalus, a condition when the brain's ventricles or cavities are filled with cerebral fluid. If the fluid doesn't drain correctly, it collects in the ventricles, which grow larger and larger, pushing and squeezing the brain against the walls of the skull and causing severe brain damage. The head is usually disproportionately large in comparison to the rest of the body. We had to go see the specialists at UC Davis, and all the follow-up scans showed enlarged ventricles. After numerous tests, the doctor sat us down in his office for a consultation.

"There is a chance," he told us gravely, "your baby could be blind, deaf, mentally impaired, all of the above, or nothing at all."

How does one process that kind of information? I was twenty weeks pregnant, a critical stage when I could still abort the baby. But I couldn't do it! In utero surgery on the fetus's brain was considered and discussed, but it was highly risky. The surgeon would install a shunt to drain cerebral fluid from the brain of the unborn baby. It is a dangerous procedure for mother and baby, so we decided against it. Pregnancy wasn't easy, and I was very frightened but prepared to deal with anything. I was on bed rest most of the time. Labor was induced when the baby's head was still small enough that delivery wouldn't cause additional brain damage. After labor had been induced, the doctor inserted a large needle into the uterus to draw amniotic fluid, which was sent to the lab in Reno. When the tests came back, they showed the baby's lungs were not yet fully developed. As that presents additional risk to the baby, labor was stopped, and I was sent home to further bed rest and to wait and wait and wait. It was nerve-racking and exhausting. I drove to the hospital every two days to run a stress test on the baby.

One day I said to my doctor, "Peter, I am done with this. I'm coming in. I want to see this baby and deal with it!" I was prepared for the worst, hoping for the best. Tom was away on business, and my parents were with me to help with our three-year-old. I drove myself to the hospital, and as soon as the nurse strapped the monitor belt on my stomach, she noticed contractions had already started. The baby and I were both ready. This was in the afternoon of June 1, 1992.

Jana was born at eight in the morning on June 2. Tom arrived just in time for her birth. It was right at the time between the hospital's night and morning shift. All the nurses from both shifts were in the delivery room. We knew many personally, thanks to our tight-knit community.

Everyone was in anxious anticipation. When Jana was born, my body went into shock, but I lay and prayed with my legs still in stirrups as I was being stitched up. I was waiting for a cry that just wouldn't come. The specialist, who was present at labor, whisked the baby away and rushed her out without even giving me a chance to see her. They took her in for a brain scan and further tests. The world around me stopped. "My baby, I need to see my baby," I kept repeating. When they finally brought her back to me, the nurse said, "Here is your beautiful, perfectly healthy baby girl."

Just a few months before my bike trip, Jana finished her master's degree in speech pathology. She is my miracle baby.

Somehow, I managed to get back to sleep after Jana's warning dream. *Thanks for the heads-up on the cows, Jana! If it weren't for you, they might have murdered me in my sleep*, I joked with my daughter in my mind.

In the morning, after cold coffee and a couple of cookies, I was back riding on the salt flats by eight, finishing an apple as I rode. Twenty more miles brought me to Ejido El Datil, a small fishing community of houses built of plywood and any other materials the people could find. It was poor by our standards, but it also had a familiar rhythm of families living and working together. Kids rode around on their rusty bikes; two young boys sat on boats cleaning fishing nets. No one was in a hurry to go anywhere. I was hungry, looking for food. Soon, I found a place with a tiny store that mainly sold cookies, chips, and other junk, but Rosa, the lady of the house, made me a brunch of three eggs and beans that I polished off with three tortillas. Heaven!

Rosa's husband sat on a bench, strumming a guitar. Their son and two grandsons were getting ready to go fishing, putting on their white rubber boots. But first, they drove off to find some gasoline for my stove. I sat and chatted with Rosa.

After fifty-two miles, I finally reached San Juanico and Scorpion Bay, home to a famous surf break. I was exhausted and famished. I set up my tent on the bluff alongside the surfers. After a cold shower, a margarita, and an excellent dinner at a nearby restaurant, I was revived again. I was in my tent by eight o'clock. My phone was dead, so I couldn't read or write, and I was soon lulled to sleep by the waves.

I was awakened suddenly by winds so powerful that I was afraid my tent was going to get blown off the bluff. Sand blasted my skin through the mesh sidewalls. *Free midnight dermabrasion procedure,* I comforted myself, trying to see something positive while eating and breathing fine sand. I prayed that I had staked down the tent down well enough that the rain fly wouldn't blow away. And then, a couple of hours later, just as quickly as it had come up, it stopped. I surrendered to the sound of the waves again.

I woke to a bright, calm morning and decided to have a rest day. I needed it badly. I had to remind myself again to stop rushing. I promised myself that I would look around and enjoy this journey. I again remembered what my father had taught me: *This is not just a bike ride to get you to the finish line. Listen! Listen to what your body is telling you. Listen to what your heart wants. You're supposed to be on a healing journey. Instead, you are killing yourself! You're never going to have a chance to do this again, ever. This is it, your lifelong dream come true. Remember what the mother abbess said: "You have to live the life you were born to live!"*

—TWENTY-FIVE—
Will the Sun Rise Again?

Oh, darling, I've been so miserable.
—Ernest Hemingway

On Tuesday, November 13, my day started early. When I unzipped my tent to take in the view from the bluff, the sky was dark red, and Sirius stared back at me. It was brighter than I'd ever seen it, just getting ready to be swallowed by the Pacific. It looked like a beacon of hope, and I was quite desperate for it. I hoped to find the strength to continue.

The fine sand had found its way into my ears, eyes, nose, sleeping bag, and everything else in my tent. Although it was not blowing as hard as it had during the night, the wind was strong enough that I didn't want to deal with the stove, mainly to avoid early morning frustration. I mixed Nescafé with cold water and headed to a nearby restaurant to recharge my phone. It was a simple place only enclosed by the walls of woven palm leaves on three sides and a palm thatched roof. The adjacent kitchen was closed, and the power shut off. So, I just sat there, staring at the ocean, waiting for the world around me to wake up. Finally, the restaurant opened, and I was able to order coffee and breakfast.

The sun came up, and with it, the strong, gusty wind returned.

By the time I finished breakfast, I was worried about my tent, unattended without my body weight to hold it down. I hurried over and was relieved it was still there. A guy later told me he had seen plenty of tents and gear fly off the cliff into the ocean below. By then, there was more than an inch of sand in my tent again. I packed everything in gusting winds as best I could and headed to town in search of a motel. I was burned out and in desperate need of rest. I passed a hotel on the main road, but it didn't look inviting. I passed another on the side street overlooking the ocean, but it looked too expensive.

Returning to the beach restaurant, I saw that they had a tiny room for rent, and even though it didn't feature a window and wasn't big enough to fit my bike into, it was a luxury.

With gratitude, I checked in and took a nap. I read. I studied maps. I looked for any inspiration to finish the trip but couldn't quite find it. When I got back on the road the next day, I hoped the journey would find me again. I hoped to find the journey I'd started. I felt like a horse that wanted to get to the barn as quickly as possible.

I also caught up with the rest of the world by watching CNN in the restaurant. California was on fire! People were dead, properties destroyed, everything gone—devastation of grand proportion! I was heartbroken. The country was nervous, the world was worried, and half an hour of watching the news filled me with dread. Politics, climate change, people just acting downright stupid and irrational. My heart was heavy with sadness.

We are on the brink of something extraordinary, more significant than humanity has ever known. We don't know it yet, and it will not come all at once. We are in a period of transformation toward something new and different. It is inevitable. Our civilization, as we know it, has peaked. There are signs all around us. And it's not the first time. The world is out of balance.

Maybe this break wasn't such a good idea after all. At least watching the news wasn't. The table next to me filled up with a bunch of local school kids who had come to celebrate their teacher's birthday. It immediately changed my somber mood. Songs, laughter, and kids drinking way too many sodas made me look on the brighter side of life again. And then I remembered the brilliant lyrics from the Monty Python song "Always Look on the Bright Side of Life," and started to whistle the refrain from the song as I walked down to the bluff to watch the surfers.

I remembered only parts of the song, so I hummed most of it, but it did help me feel much better as music and comedy always does. I wondered if life really was just a piece of shit in the end.

My tiny room was next to the restaurant, which closed at nine o'clock, but a group of local guys played cards late into the night, talking and laughing very loudly and drinking beer and tequila. I tried to ignore the noise. My ears were stuffed with earplugs, but I just couldn't sleep. I looked at my phone, and it was one in the morning. I got out of bed and headed to the bathroom, which was outside next to the restaurant. I slammed the door of my room on purpose and angrily sent dagger eyes in their direction. I instantly regretted that. It was maybe just a tad over the top, but I was furious. It was dark, so I hoped they hadn't seen the angry look I'd cast in their direction. I realized I probably shouldn't have done that. These guys were drunk, and there was no one else around. I hurried into the bathroom and stayed in there for a long time, listening. I finally heard car doors slamming before they drove off. I was relieved but made sure I locked the door behind me. The windowless room was so small it felt suffocating because the air couldn't move around.

I tossed and turned all night, checking the time that seemed to have stopped. I wanted the night to end, but I didn't want the morning to arrive either. Morning meant departure, and I wasn't ready for it. I started examining the maps at six o'clock and was filled with dread. I was looking for a shortcut to get to La Paz and considered skipping riding through the mission section of the route. I grabbed a cup of coffee when the restaurant opened and walked to the bluff. Surfers were out ripping the waves already. It was immediately apparent to me what to do.

"I'm staying another day to have a proper rest," I said aloud to myself.

The previous day had been windy and cold and miserable.

And just like that, by my act of surrender, everything was clear again. I knew exactly where, when, and how I was going to continue my ride.

Scorpion Bay includes six different right-hand point breaks on which rides can last for a long time. On a mellow day, the surf is suited for beginners. I went for a refreshing swim. The water must have been around seventy degrees. I caught a perfect wave body surfing, and it brought me all the way to shore. But I scraped my thigh on a razor-sharp piece of coral, giving it a nice cut, one more thing to worry about.

Watching the surfers made me happy. Some guys and gals looked effortless, dancing on the waves riding their boards; others were beginners, and then there were fathers with their little boys and girls on the same surfboard. One father even rode with a son and a dog on his board. A crusty old guy surfed with a goat! I was tempted to beg a board off someone to try to catch a wave, but I was quite content just sitting and watching.

I was so glad I'd decided to stay another day. My mother would often say to me that everything happened for a reason. At dusk, I was in my tiny room looking over the maps when I heard someone say, "Do you know Alenka? She's from Tahoe. She's riding a bike."

I bolted out of bed and was out of my mind excited to see our neighbors from Tahoe, Tom and Carol Carter, standing right outside my door. They had been traveling down here for the last three weeks and had been in touch with Jim via text. Somehow the timing had worked out perfectly. We could not have planned to meet, even if we'd wanted to. Had I left in the morning as intended, we would have missed each other by less than a day.

I never tire of Tom's energetic stories about skiing and mountain-eering adventures around the world, from teaching Nordic skiing at Von Trapp family lodge in Vermont, to a National Geographic-sponsored photo assignment trip of the first-ever midwinter traverse of New Zealand's Southern Alps, to climbing Yosemite's El Capitan thirteen times. Thirteen times! Can you believe that? He is a legend in the climbing and skiing community and a world-known avalanche expert. I met Tom in the spring of 1988 at Ruby Mountains, where he worked as a heli-ski guide for thirty winters. We sat at the restaurant drinking margaritas, and I was plenty drunk after my second. The stories of adventures kept flowing, refilling my emotional cup, bringing me closer to home.

As we said goodnight, I felt truly reenergized and ready to continue with my journey. In the morning, I took off at first light. As I passed their Eurovan Westfalia camper parked on the bluff, we said our goodbyes, and I rode toward La Purísima.

Sierras Gigantas, Missiones, here I come!

The very sound of its name sounded beautiful and inviting.

And more.

La Purísima promised further purification of my soul.

—TWENTY-SIX—
Seeing in Color

The universe talks to itself:
We are its tongue and ears,
Its words and silences.

—Octavio Paz

There was something about the pattern of my perceptions when I first arrived at an unfamiliar place. At first, I was guarded against the unknown. As I learned more about my new environment, I began to build a relationship with it.

I left San Juanico on Thursday, November 15. After thirty-six miles on a mix of dirt, rock, and ankle-deep soft sand, I found myself on a remote and lonely road with the temperature hovering around a hundred degrees. Slowly, I descended to the valley of La Purísima and crossed a river. A river in the desert looked odd, out of place, unfamiliar, yet it was a welcome sight. It was such a striking contrast to the barren, hot desert that I'd just ridden across. A blue heron and a huge osprey noisily flew off, startled by my arrival. The moving water was clear, fresh, and inviting, unlike other rivers I'd passed that were murky, bug-infested, and polluted by cow poop.

I was just starting to take off my shoes and shorts to take a dip when two dirt bike riders appeared from the direction I'd ridden.

They had picked up my water bottle along the way, which I hadn't realized had dropped off the bike. I needed to do something to stop losing water bottles! I was angry with myself. I found an extra rubber strap and tied the bottle securely back onto the dropouts holding the rear wheel. I added a couple more zip ties, but I only had two left, as they kept breaking off while the bike rattled down bumpy roads. It was obviously not the best setup.

Fortunately, one of the guys lived in Los Barriles, an hour south by car from my final destination, and was familiar with the roads ahead. As we compared where we were going, he gave me useful information about what I should expect.

"The section between Constitution and La Paz is long, rocky, and very difficult, with lots of climbing," he said, "but you'll also be riding through beautiful, cake-layered canyons. Make sure you have enough water and food for that section. Not much along that road till you are almost in La Paz."

I thanked him, and the two of them rode off.

I rode the remainder of the distance to town on pavement. A short climb led me through a narrow canyon with steep walls dotted with white goats that looked like the first snowflakes of winter. The valley opened into a beautiful date palm oasis. The canyon walls were topped by a volcano shaped like a sombrero. I rode through town on streets lined by empty, dilapidated buildings with broken windows that had once served a variety of businesses. I passed small farmhouses, a playground, a plaza, a mission, and a boarded-up hotel. The town looked rundown and deserted, yet there were signs of revival as well.

On the other end, a store buzzed with people and activity. Trucks lined up, and people milled about: vaqueros with their white cowboy hats, women with kids holding onto their legs with little ones resting on their hips. The history of Baja ranching and its legendary vaqueros dates to the arrival of the Spanish in 1519. Cattle and horses were imported from Spain, and new landowners trained native people the riding and roping skills that became legendary. The roots of the Alta California cowboy or buckaroo started right here in the heart of Baja.

Life on these ranches hasn't changed much. Many ranchos are far removed from the rest of civilization, and traditions are still passed down to the next generations as they have been for over three hundred years. It remains the Wild West and the frontier in many ways, untouched by the outside world. The ranches are not easily accessible by car, and many can only be reached on the backs of horses, mules, and burros. Generations of families live together in what we might consider primitive dirt-floor huts and cook over open fires, which burn day and night. Everyone has chores, and much of their hard life depends on water, which can be extremely scarce. This was another reason I wanted to ride my bike through remote areas. I wanted to experience the old ways of life in Baja before it was too late.

A food stand in front of the store offered tacos, hot dogs, and *tortas*, a delicious Mexican sandwich roll, toasted, smothered with spicy mayo, and loaded with shredded pork. A line of people waited for their food. Several local guys quickly surrounded The Beast, admiring it, which always made me feel uneasy.

I was hungry, and I needed a cold beer. I felt like I would insult people if I locked the bike in front of everyone. By trusting the people of this beautiful village, I hoped to show them my respect. That was the "code of the road" I wanted to live by. I recalled the conversation I'd had with Marion just the day before I crossed into Mexico. Given a chance, we are all honest creatures. I went to the store to grab a cold beer and prayed that the bike would be there when I returned. Of course, it was. I sat at the only table with the vaqueros, and I learned that this kind of activity happens only twice a month, on the fifteenth and at the end of the month when farmers come to the village from the surrounding ranches to sell their goat cheese, which was then distributed to cities in Baja and the mainland. It was a cheese renowned for its purity and quality. Farmers bought food and other necessities and mingled for a bit before returning to their ranchos in the hills. The store was the central gathering spot. By then, my relationship with the place had already deepened. It had a human pulse. Humans are not solitary animals. We are codependent, social animals who need interaction.

After a delicious torta, a refreshing beer, and conversations with local people, I rode to the campground I'd passed at the beginning of town. My perception of the village had changed as I'd adapted to this new environment. I felt like I was in a different dimension. I saw and smelled and heard in color. Human nature seeks familiarity and comfort and some constancy. I had been battling the new, the uncertain, and my solitary state for almost two months. Discovering new places, meeting new people, and speaking in a new language is an astonishing experience. It requires constant adaptation and readjustment from what is expected and what is real. It requires ingenuity and resourcefulness. It is incredibly rewarding, yet exhausting, as you must continually be on guard. It is extraordinarily difficult, both physically and emotionally, and it often takes a toll on your mental state from which you then fight your way back to rebalance. I needed a rest from it all and was ready for some stability; I was ready to be in a familiar and secure environment surrounded by people I knew and loved. I was ready to go *home*! In a curious way, the closer I came to the end of my pilgrimage, the more I longed for home.

When I returned to the campground and met the owner of the property, I ended up splurging and rented a room in a cabana for twenty-five dollars. It doesn't seem like much, but as I wasn't traveling with much cash on me, I was getting seriously low on money. I had to have enough for food and to get me to Ciudad Concepcion, where there was a bank. I had just a few more pesos left. I hadn't had a hot shower since I'd left San Ignacio several days before. My body melted as hot water caressed my tired muscles. I met the owner's husband, and they were both delightful people. Their place was beautiful, and they were building more cabanas, which were rustic and very tastefully done, as was the campground by the river. They were very proud of their son, who was an architect, and it showed. In the morning, I got a tour of the wine cave and lush gardens where vines that arrived with the first Spanish missionaries were thriving.

I took my time leaving, but not before I promised I would return for the wine festival. I imagined a return with Jim. I missed sharing with him these exciting things I was experiencing, yet I wondered how different it would be when we returned. Would we find it intriguing and be able to appreciate it, like I did at that moment?

I rode the dirt road along the river out of town toward San Isidro, another palm oasis. It then climbed in and out of many drainage basins. I passed several goat ranches along the way. Time had stopped there decades before. Homes were built mainly with materials found in and around the area. Goats roamed freely, and they were adorable. I wanted a goat! I didn't know what I'd do with it, but I wanted one. They do make great pets. I wondered what our golden retriever, Monty, would think of that.

On a high plateau, the sweet smell of blooming yellow flowers saturated the air. They had carpeted the ground after a rain a few weeks earlier. I closed my eyes and listened to the symphony of millions of bees gathering pollen and honey. Yellow-and-white butterflies darted from one tiny flower to another. Nature was hard at work and in perfect harmony.

When I arrived at Scorpion Bay, I'd hit a wall. I studied maps to find the shortest, quickest, straightest way to La Ventana Bay. I seriously contemplated skipping the Mission part of the ride. I knew there would be a lot of climbing involved and minimal supply spots along the route. Physically as well as mentally, I was exhausted. During my much-needed, two-day break, I recovered and learned more about the path and places ahead; it gave me the courage and energy to continue. I was so glad I did!

A steep descent finally dropped me at San Jose De Comondú. A lush palm oasis lay below, and the town was larger than I'd anticipated. I hoped there would be a place to camp and get a bite to eat. If not, I'd figure something out as I always did. The dirt road turned into cobblestone, and I passed an older couple. They were nicely dressed and heading to town. It was Friday night, so there was likely something happening. I greeted them as I passed, and they greeted me back. I was already past them when the man yelled after me in Spanish, "Where are you from, Germany?"

I stopped, turned around and answered, "No, I am actually from Slovenia."

That got the conversation going.

I asked, "Is there a place to sleep and eat in town?" Surely, they would know.

They looked at each other, and the woman said, "Well, why don't you just come and stay at our house?" I couldn't believe this "*¿Estas Seguro?*" Are you sure? I asked, amazed at my luck again.

"*Por supuesto!*" They both exclaimed enthusiastically. Of course! Warm evening light shone in Omar's dark brown eyes full of kindness, as he lovingly tugged at his wife's elbow.

We all turned around and walked back to their home. Rosalva and Omar were retired and lived in La Paz but spent a lot of time in Comondú village. They reminded me of my parents. Rosalva showed me where to park The Beast, pointed me to a room with three beds, and told me to pick one. I felt like Goldilocks. They fed me a bowl of delicious vegetable soup, a quesadilla made with local goat cheese and beans, and dates for dessert. Then Rosalva pointed me to a bathroom. After I'd showered, we walked out to the central plaza. The town was anticipating a big wine festival on the weekend. We listened to live music on the plaza for an hour or so in the company of a handful of locals. It was fun for a while, but I was tired. Luckily, they were as well. We headed back to the house, had some tea brewed from fresh citrus leaves, and I retired to my cozy bed to a much-deserved rest. My stomach was full, and my heart was bursting, I had a safe bed. Life was complete at that moment.

And I was so close to La Ventana that I could practically taste it.

—TWENTY-SEVEN—
Trouble on the Horizon

*I want to stand as close to the edge as I can without going
over. Out on the edge you see all the kinds of things you
can't see from the center.*
—Kurt Vonnegut, Jr.

What goes down must come up again. Just as the road steeply
descended into this lush oasis, it climbed steeply out of it. My
breakfast wanted to come up as well, and long, loud burps competed with the sounds of the birds keeping me company on that fine
Saturday morning. It was November 17, and I wished I could stay
for the wine festivities. People were arriving from near and far. But I
didn't want to overstay a kind invitation and impose on Rosalva and
Omar. Plus, my heart wanted to keep going. I needed to finish. It was
getting more and more difficult for me to think about how much Jim,
my kids, and the rest of my family and friends were worrying about
me.

As I moved through town, I wondered how the first explorers
of Baja had managed to discover this place in 1684, tucked so far
away in the mountains. I wondered what had possessed the Jesuits
to build such a large mission in this valley back in 1708. To colo-
nize the area, Spain was awarded the land by the Catholic Church.

The Jesuits started to build the outposts and introduced European livestock, fruits, and vegetables to be self-supporting as they were in such remote parts. Water, of course, was the key to existence, but so was labor to cultivate crops and tend livestock. Several indigenous nomadic native tribes like the Monqui, Cochimí, and Guayacura had lived in this area for thousands of years before the Spanish explorers and Jesuits arrived. Unaccustomed to living in permanent locations, they often ran away to escape forced labor and efforts of conversion to the strict religious practices of the Catholic Church. Their numbers were soon drastically reduced as they succumbed to foreign diseases like smallpox and measles.

There are many locations in Baja, several that I'd passed, that contain large cave and rock paintings. They house drawings made from powdered rock pigments that have resisted time, preserving at least some of the story in often elaborate and abstract expressions of the native peoples of this land. I frequently felt the strong presence of the ghosts of the past while riding in these remote mountains.

A rough road meandered up and down, passing several more goat ranches. As I descended into another drainage basin at exactly 11:11, I turned the corner, and before me loomed a sheer wall with a steep road carved into it, zigzagging back and forth. Well, Beast, what choice do we have? Let's put on a brave face and grind this one out. We've done it many times, and we can do it again. We have water, we have time, we are well-fed, and we have an extra reserve of love from two strangers who, in a short time, became our new friends.

That morning, over coffee sweetened by delicious local honey, Rosalva and I discussed the secret to her happy, loving marriage. She married Omar when she was sixteen and he was twenty-six. I asked her what had made the relationship last.

She answered, "Love, of course, is the secret!"

"Yes, but what is love?" I asked. "We always say *love*, but what does that mean in real life, in everyday marriage?"

"Love is taking care of my husband," she said, and then got up to pour Omar another cup of coffee. It was not a submissive or servile act. He rose slowly after he finished his cup, thanked her, and kissed her on her cheek.

She continued, "Love is taking care of our four daughters when they were growing up in La Paz. Love is keeping the home nice and tidy and stress-free for my husband. Love is mutual respect, tolerance, patience, and avoiding quick judgment. Love is singing and dancing together."

And they did. Their favorite song came on, which they have danced to for nearly fifty years in their long life together. They danced in their kitchen at breakfast right in front of me. I quietly watched as these two lovely people, in love after so many years, waltzed around the room. All I wanted in that moment was to get home into my husband's embrace so we could dance our own dance.

Riding at the far edge of the rocky road rutted by torrential rains, I was immersed in that scene. I imagined that Jim and I would soon be dancing under the starry night sky, with soft music playing from an old-fashioned gramophone. I imagined a piano, clarinet, and violins guiding us through the perfectly synchronized dance moves, as we dreamily gazed into each other's eyes.

Jim and I don't actually own a gramophone, and setting a romantic mood is not on Jim's high-priority list. But that doesn't mean I can't daydream about dancing with him, imagining his sky-blue eyes holding my gaze again for a few long seconds under the purple night sky, with twinkling crystals blinking down on us.

I was so immersed in this fantasy that I failed to notice where the bike was going.

My front wheel caught a sharp-edged rock, which suddenly appeared out of nowhere, hiding in plain sight among the other rocks surrounding it. The wheel veered to the right, sliding off the edge of the trail, and then the rest of the bike, heavy and unruly as a stubborn mule, followed down into the abyss. Having absolutely no control over the bike nor my destiny, I was quickly gaining speed, as it was so steep that the brakes did nothing. The Beast and I did the best we could avoiding several large boulders coming at us with a deadly speed. Soon the battle was lost. We bounced off one large, beautifully shaped piece of smooth granite boulder, polished by centuries of erosion and waiting just for us. We sideswiped it and flipped into the air, flying toward our final resting place. When I was aware of my surroundings again, I was trapped underneath the crushing weight of the bike, unable to move.

"Ahhhh!" I groaned as a sharp pain rushed through my right leg and arm as if the spoke of the wheel had gone right through my body, splitting it in half. I was lying on a bed of rocks, and the small cactus I'd landed on was poking me in the ribs. My head, pointing downhill on a steep and rocky slope, was wedged between two boulders. I just lay there breathing slow, shallow, quiet breaths as if I didn't dare to disturb the silence.

Looking at the Baja sky, I didn't want to move. Puffy white clouds floated above me. A whale passed, looking down on me, and then it metamorphosed into a rabbit. I could just stay like that and be the little girl I once was, lying in the meadow of tall grasses behind our home and looking at a church of Saint Peter atop a green hill. I closed my eyes. I wanted to go to sleep. "Take me home," I whispered to the whale above. I wanted to go home. I was suddenly startled. My mind screamed, *Get up, you dummy!*

When I opened my eyes, I could see vultures circling above. Now the cloud was just a blob, spinning, stretching, and dissolving. Slowly I dragged myself from under the heavy bike, groaning with pain. I sat next to The Beast, checking my cuts and bruises. My knee and elbow were bleeding, and my head had a nice gash right by my ear, but, apart from my pride, it appeared nothing was broken. My head throbbed. I looked as if a puma had attacked me.

By then, I was hours away from any help. It took a tremendous effort to drag The Beast back onto the trail, bags and water holders hanging loosely. I collected my gear, which lay scattered in the path of destruction. I limped along for a while and then got back on the bike to slowly push my way to the top of the climb.

When I finally reached the top of the canyon, I had to fix my water bottle holders, which had broken when we went tumbling, with the last of my zip ties. I laid the bike down in the middle of the road. No cars pass by here, but wouldn't you know it. Just as I was in the middle of my repairs, and still licking my wounds, feeling sorry for myself, a jeep came bouncing along. I had to drag The Beast and all my scattered stuff off the narrow road.

The vehicle slowed, and I was introduced to an older gentleman who was traveling from Loreto to San Juan de Comondú to the wine festival. We chatted for a bit and exchanged information as to what conditions were ahead on the road. "You sure you're okay?" he asked. "You look pretty beat up!"

"I'm fine, thanks, just a bit sore!"

He handed me a bottle of water. "Here, wash your cuts a bit!"

I described Rosalva and Omar and asked him to give them my best. As he took off, I got back to fixing the bike. I loved having the whole quiet place to myself again.

I continued riding the rough roads, meandering up and down with no end in sight. I tried to ignore the heat, which hovered around a hundred degrees. I tried to ignore the throbbing in my head and limbs. I was surrounded by steep mountains covered in low brush and granite boulders as I rode through picturesque canyons that held secrets of many lives lived here before me. They led me to San Javier, yet another beautiful mission town. A family was renting out a couple of small, primitive cabanas they had built in their backyard. Sitting in their courtyard, the whole family greeted me, "*¿Sola? Sin esposo?*"

They were aghast that I was traveling alone without a husband.

Once again, my mere appearance was a shock to the traditional way for women to travel and even be in the world. Soon, I met cousins, sisters, sisters-in-law, husbands, a grandfather, and the youngest member of the family, a precocious, chubby four-year-old granddaughter. The mother of the house showed me to my cabana built of thin plywood.

I mixed a bottle of electrolyte drink and lay wrapped in my down quilt on a bunk. I had no appetite, which left me more than a bit concerned. I still had eighty-two miles to reach Ciudad Constitucion, and from there, 215 more miles to La Ventana. I studied what was still ahead. Resupply opportunities would be very limited. My notes said the route would be hot, low country, followed by steep and rocky passes. I could not possibly get sick on this last stretch. It was still one of the most challenging and strenuous sections of the Baja Divide. I'd come too far. Begging my body to cooperate, I nibbled on the last of the chips, forcing them down with electrolyte water. I knew I should eat something more nutritious, but I couldn't even think of food.

I was also down to my last peso banknotes and some change in my pockets, so reaching a town with a bank was crucial. I had even used up my hidden emergency twenty-dollar bill. My night was restless, every inch of my body aching.

On Sunday morning, the whole family gathered early to prepare a traditional meal of a goat's head slowly steamed underground. While singing and dancing, the women chopped vegetables that would steam with the goat's head. The men prepared the fire, but they mostly sat around waiting for the women to serve them coffee. Beer would follow soon.

I sat in their kitchen, feeling like a mangled cat that had barely survived a fight. I watched the action and interaction among different generations. Earlier, I'd told the grandmother that I'd been having stomach troubles that started the night before. It's amazing, and I felt lucky that this was the first time on the whole trip I'd been sick, but it seemed that the trip was catching up with me. The cramping continued throughout the night, and now I was sitting in a strange kitchen feeling miserable. The women consulted each other, then one of the daughters ran out to the yard and returned with some green leaves that the grandmother steeped in hot water for ten minutes. The tea tasted bitter. Whatever was still in my stomach wanted to come up. They assured me it was good for me. While I sat there sipping the remedy, I wondered about all the good and all the bad that "progress" brings.

For centuries people were able to live off the land, but the chubby four-year-old was munching on Doritos Flamas for breakfast. I went for a walk by the mission through the ancient growth of olive trees, a citrus grove, and grapevines. Several olive trees were more than four hundred years old. The original trees and grapevines were planted by Jesuits in the eighteenth century. Fertile ground and fresh water provided a beautiful setting. This mission location was the first where grapes were grown and wine produced in the Californias. A freshwater spring a kilometer away was connected to the gardens by a stone aqueduct. An elaborate watering system was still visible and had been largely preserved.

People arrived from surrounding villages as far as Loreto, twenty-two miles away, for a one o'clock mass. I entered the magnificent stone church. The walls were as much as seven feet wide, and despite the down jacket I was wearing, I shivered in the chill. The heavy wooden door shut behind me, and everything went dark and quiet. I always felt awkward going through the motions of crossing and kneeling when I entered the church. But I liked the ritual of it, so I obliged.

I sat down in a second-row pew, leaned my head against the wood from the bench in front of me, and closed my eyes. Feeling the cool wood pressing against my forehead, I said a prayer my grandma taught me, which I knew only in my native Slovene language: *Oče naš, ki si v nebesih . . .* Our father who art in heaven . . ."

I got lost halfway. I didn't know what I was praying for, except that it made me think of my very devout grandmothers, Mama Hani and Mama Mira. It connected me with them and the home I had left so long ago. I prayed for a safe passage just in case someone was actually listening: "I am tired. I am hurt. I am sick. I am so close, but I need strength to get through this last part. Get me home safely."

I opened my eyes, and a beautiful sliver of light was falling through the glass windows across the slick stone floor. I followed it outside. I was out of money, and I barely had enough to pay for the night's stay by collecting all the coins I had scattered in various pockets and a small bag tied to the frame on my bike. I didn't have a peso left. I went and said goodbye to my host family. My stomach and I were at war. I couldn't eat anything. I wanted to cinch my Velcro belt tighter, as my shorts were falling down while I walked, but I had lost so much weight on the journey there was no more adhesive left on my belt.

I saddled The Beast and rode out of town like an old-fashioned cowgirl.

The ride meandered along the San Javier River. My aching body slowly warmed, and I kept trying to get comfortable on my seat. I passed beautiful working ranches, rode through picturesque canyons, and crossed the river many times. There were cave paintings in the mountains about an hour's climb from the road. I was tempted but had absolutely no extra energy. My sole focus was to get to Ciudad Constitucion. Again, I made a mental note to return to explore the area, rich in natural beauty and ancient history, with Jim. This way, I felt he was traveling along with me all the time and urging me on. The Beast received a much-needed bath as we rode through water a couple of feet deep several times. He was quite dusty and had started to make squeaking sounds. I had to stop to lube his chain. Riding through water and sand took its toll. I hadn't treated it in a couple of days.

"I'm sorry, Beast," I said, "I'm starting to neglect you, but I'm just not feeling like myself!"

Although there wasn't much climbing, progress was slow on the river rock road, and many sections were sandy. The scenery was spectacular: vegetation lush, the cardón forests beautiful. I passed a vaquero on a spirited black horse, and I felt bad that I'd spooked him. The horse started rearing as I passed, and the vaquero used his expert skills to back off the trail and away from me.

In the heat of the day, I took a dip in a clear, refreshing pool surrounded by smooth, white granite boulders. The shock of cold water revived me. I swam fully dressed so I could keep cool for a while riding in wet clothes. As I crossed the riverbed with running water for the last time, a rancher passed me in an old beat-up pickup. He stopped, and we talked for a while. He was on his way back from visiting his brother. He owned a ranch called Agua Bonita. And it really was a beautiful place. Water was everywhere, a deep emerald.

He was a genuinely nice man, and he wished me a very safe journey as he pulled away.

Just before sunset, I found a perfect camp spot by a dry riverbed. The ground was covered in fine, soft sand, and there was plenty of dry wood to build a fire. As I was setting up the tent, a curious hummingbird danced around me. He landed on a branch and just sat there watching me for a long time, tipping his tiny head from side to side. His feathers were a brilliant rainbow of green and scarlet. Crickets commenced their evening prayer song, and the wind sang in the tops of the trees all around me. A thin layer of clouds enshrouded the moon, and all was peaceful and quiet. There is something extraordinary about being alone in the desert, next to a fire surrounded by all that magic. Open space, open mind. It was a shame that the stars were hiding behind the clouds, but you can't wish for what's not there. So often we long for what we don't have, and we fail to fully engage with and enjoy what is there, right in front of us, right then at that very moment in time. That moment was precious, and it would never repeat itself. I was at peace, but my stomach was doing flips.

I sipped on a cup of tea, hoping it would sooth the pain in my twisted guts. I realized it was the first night that I was not being eaten alive by mosquitoes. A few bugs flew around attracted by the fire, but I could safely say that I'd had a perfect day followed by a beautiful evening, and, hopefully, I would have a restful night.

By the morning, my stomach troubles returned with a vengeance. Shooting pains caused by intense cramping traveled throughout my ravaged body. I had to rush out of my tent, fumbling with the zipper in the dark, and dig a hole in the sand just in the nick of time. Whatever food was still in me, gushed out from both ends, and was now buried in the sand on the banks of the dry riverbed. I pinched my loose skin on my bicep, and the skin just remained pinched.

Dehydration scared the shit out of me. I was losing not just weight, but also muscle mass. My skin and clothes hung loosely on my bony body. I took the diarrhea meds my doctor friend had prescribed and prayed they would start working before I lost any more fluids. The tea that grandma prepared for me the day before had lost its magic.

I struggled to ride the last miles on sandy and rocky, but flat, roads. The road was quiet, the scenery unremarkable. Or maybe I just didn't see the beauty in it any longer. I was too preoccupied with how I felt. The decision had been made for me. I was crushed. I crossed the main highway at Ley Federal #1, and rode the last twenty-five miles through citrus groves, arriving at the big agricultural city of Constitution utterly spent, barely able to balance my bike, which had grown heavier with every mile. I needed to catch a bus to La Paz. If my condition worsened, I could get myself into serious trouble. The last of the energy squeezed out of me with every drop of water that escaped each pore and cavity. I needed to recover overnight in La Paz, so I could at least ride the last leg of the trip to La Ventana. I found the bus station in the center of town, and I was in luck. The bus was on schedule to leave in an hour. I was able to buy a ticket with a credit card. I sat by the bike on the ground, eating salty chips and drinking electrolytes when the bus arrived.

"No room for the bike!" said the driver, hardly looking at me as he smoked and talked with a buddy at the station.

He pointed to the opened compartments, which were all full. His assistant was shoving the last of the bags into tight spaces.

This wasn't happening!

I was so desperate to get on the bus that I couldn't possibly give up hope.

"But I have a ticket!" I pulled it out of my pocket and showed it to him while giving him a pleading look. I took the front wheel off and just stood forlornly by the bus hoping for mercy. The driver's young assistant opened the third compartment, which held the bus's spare tire. The Beast fit in perfectly.

I welcomed riding the bus across the incredibly long, flat stretch between Ciudad Constitucion and La Paz. Just thinking about not having to ride across this vast plateau, dehydrated and sick with diarrhea and cramping, unable to eat, not knowing where I'd sleep or if I had enough water, made me so happy. It was better I skipped that part for the time being. I promised myself I would return to finish this portion when I recovered.

As the cardóns and palo verdes flew by, I leaned my forehead against the cool glass and thought how my journey was now coming to an end, knowing it would be impossible to repeat. It was my journey alone, in that time and space. Even if you had traveled with me, it would have been a completely different kind of trip for you. It would have been entirely your own experience. Even if I turned around right then and started the ride all over again, I would have an entirely new ride. At that moment, I realized I would never be able to advise anyone for or against it. If anyone were to ask upon my return, I would be obligated to say, "You have to find your own journey. We all do."

The bus arrived in the city in the dark. John Steinbeck would be rolling in his grave if he were to see the sprawling city of La Paz today. Long gone are the days of rowing in dugout canoes by native Indian Pericú and Guaycura tribes who once lived on the shores of that beautiful bay.

I've been coming to La Paz for over twenty years, and it has grown exponentially during that time. My surroundings were bright and loud. I was not used to all the commotion, all those people around me. I felt lonelier than when I was all alone camping in the desert surrounded by mountains and stars, days away from everyone and everything. I felt more scared as well because I was surrounded by so many people. I was nervous at the bank getting cash. I was scared walking to the cockroach motel on a narrow, dimly lit street. I felt suffocated in the cinderblock room without a window for fresh air. I longed for the open road, and my arrival in the big city felt anticlimactic.

The bathroom smelled like raw sewage. I'd rather smell cow poop. I finally discovered that the room had a fan that ran at five speeds. I turned it to number one, which I assumed was the slowest. The room wanted to take off like a jet-powered helicopter. I turned it "down" to five. Now I could breathe. I spread out my sleeping quilt, inflated my own pillow, and hoped for some sleep. I also hoped the meds would take effect and my night would be peaceful enough that I could regain enough energy to ride home to La Ventana in the morning.

The night found me restless. The room was stuffy, my stomach churned all night, and I was a bundle of nerves tossing and turning on an uncomfortable bed, my guts in knots. I killed a couple more roaches in the corner of the room, and I couldn't wait to take off in the morning. I awoke early and impatiently waited for first light to arrive. I squeezed The Beast through the narrow door of my cell into the courtyard, leaning the bike against the low garden wall to lube the chain. While I was spinning the pedal, I cut my hand on the greasy, dusty chain ring. It hurt like hell, and my hand was bleeding. "Get me out of here!" I muttered out loud.

I rode downhill through a narrow alley and back to the Malecon. The road was barricaded for an event, and though it was still early, I was greeted by people and loud music blasting through big speakers. The Bay of La Paz was bathing in early morning sunlight.

"¿Qué pasa?" What is going on? I asked two policemen directing traffic.

"Well, today is November twentieth, and it is Mexican Independence Day. We are preparing for the big parade," they told me.

Of course! I'd completely forgotten what day it was. And what a parade! Groups of kids from different schools dressed in matching outfits performed dance routines they had undoubtedly practiced for months. They were followed by sports teams and, at the end, by a young army, police, and fire cadets. Such a joyous and colorful occasion! As I stood on the bench taking photos of the kids warming up for their performance, a woman's voice wafted through the crowd. "Good morning, honey!" I looked down, and a woman on a bike was smiling back at me.

"I recognize you," she said.

"You do?" I replied, incredulous.

"Yeah, I followed your blog. Congratulations! You've made it!"

Somehow Leslie, whom I'd never met before, had found and followed my blog, which I posted on occasion with Mateja's help to keep my family and friends informed of my progress. I felt like a mini celebrity. I was in La Paz, Mexico, and this woman knew about me and my ride. It felt a bit surreal. Was this really a bigger deal than I was giving myself credit for? Anyone could do this if they really wanted to. I've always loved the lyrics of "The Real Thing" by Kenny Loggins from his 1991 album, *Leap of Faith*.

I had played that song so often on my CD in the car with my kids that it was worn down and skipping in many places. In the song, Loggins sings to his daughter and his boys that even though he and his wife had divorced, love should teach you joy, and not an imitation. His song makes it achingly clear how much he still believes in love and how we should never compromise that feeling because it is at the heart of life.

My relationship with this song is deeply personal. The famous singer had saved my daughter Jana from the bottom of a pool when we met on a ski trip in Lake Louise, Canada. We were sitting in the hot tub, and one-year-old Jana crawled away from us unnoticed. A few years later, when we visited Kenny and his family in Santa Barbara, he and I discussed how important real and honest love was. By then I was struggling in my marriage to Tom. This song helped me to understand how I needed to end my own broken relationship. Now, here in La Paz, which means Peace, I could perhaps feel at peace at last, because I had allowed my boat to sail out to sea.

Leslie and I rode along with the parade for the length of the Malecon and parted ways at the end where I turned toward the mountains. I was led out of town by loud music and high fives from kids of all ages.

The road out of La Paz gently climbed for fifteen miles over a pass. I reached the twenty-two-kilometer marker and was suddenly overwhelmed by a flood of conflicting emotions. I cried all the way until the road began its descent to La Ventana Bay. I pulled over to gather my senses and to take in the views. I was not there yet, and I told myself, "Pay attention now, Alenka! You're on the road with cars going by. You've come too far to do something stupid. Don't let your guard down until it's over. Cross the finish line, and then you can cry all you want!"

My own advice to myself was exactly what I had coached my kids on the ski team for so many years. "Don't celebrate until you cross the finish line!" I exhorted them. "Olympic medals have been lost that way."

At the bottom of a four-mile-long downhill, the road turned left for another seven miles to La Ventana. I could taste the glory of the finish line now! The words *The thrill of victory, the agony of defeat* rang in my ears. My countryman Vinko Bogataj, who lives in the neighboring village of Lesce, became famous for his 1970 Oberstdorf ski jump crash. For years it was an opening sequence to ABC's *Wide World of Sports*. I wanted to feel the thrill of victory, not be squashed by a car at the end of my journey. I rode against the wind, and I saw many kites flying over the bay. They looked like colorful butterflies caught on long strings, pulling kite surfers across the water. I couldn't wait to fly across the ocean myself on my own kiteboard, attached by ninety-foot-long lines to a kite that pulled me across the waves.

When I finally arrived at La Ventana, the first person I ran into was our friend Jerry from Tahoe. We hugged, and we both started crying.

"Jim told me you were on the way. He texted me just a little while ago. He feels bad he's not here. He wanted you to be welcomed by someone, so here we are."

I was overjoyed to be greeted by a friend and to see familiar faces after such a long time on the lonely road. "Dinner at Las Palmas at six. The whole family will be there," He exclaimed and drove off, pulling a U-turn toward La Ventana village. "You're almost home!" He waved and called out the window as he drove past me. Jerry's two little girls looked at me curiously from the back seat of the car, waving.

There were only a few more miles left to ride to my house. Everything was coming into focus. Every house I passed I recognized. Everything was familiar. The familiar felt so good. I recognized people driving and waved at them.

I am here! I wanted to scream. *Can you believe it?*

No one noticed. Everyone kept going their own way, doing their everyday things.

I made it! I survived! I just rode more than two thousand miles on my freaking bike! I wanted to tell everyone when I arrived at Oscarito's convenience store.

I wanted to celebrate. I wanted *some* kind of recognition!

Finally, I simply leaned my dusty bike against the wall of the dimly lit store.

Inside, I walked around in a daze, looking at all the stuff on the shelves. I picked up a large avocado, tomato, a large golden yellow papaya, big juicy white onion. I could now buy all this and make fresh salsa. I could cook a real meal in a big, heavy cast-iron skillet on a real stove, which would light up and stay lit without my cursing at it! I could cook for my whole family and invite friends, and we could sit at a real table, on real chairs, and eat from real plates again.

The owner of the grocery store, whom I've known for years, was at the counter, and she greeted me with a big smile when I came over with my one can of beer.

"*¿Solo una?*" she asked, laughing. Only one?

"*¡Si, solo una por ahora!*" Yes, just one beer for now.

I just had to do something to mark the occasion. I sat on a half wall in front of the store in the shade, leaning against the post and letting the beer cool me down. I closed my eyes, trying to just take it in. What did I feel? I knew I should have felt something. I didn't know what I was expecting, but certainly it was something more than just sitting in front of Oscarito's market, drinking beer by myself, surrounded by a pack of stray dogs sniffing the bags on my bike for food. I shooed the dogs and got back on my bike to ride the last mile on a dirt road in a daze and slightly tipsy from an unfinished beer.

Where was Jim? I so wanted him to be here, to greet me, to embrace me, and for once to say out loud, "I am so proud of you!" I understood that a deep part of Jim was angry with me for leaving him to worry about me. I'd lived with it every mile of my journey. It troubled me deeply, leaving me questioning why. Why do I cause such pain to the man who loves me with all his heart? He doesn't show it in a way that is often expected of him, but I know he is also terrified of losing me. I can't explain these actions of mine and most likely I never will be able to. Do I regret going on this journey? I do not. My need, drive, and desire to do something for myself, by myself was stronger than the obligations I was made to believe I needed to follow. How many men leave their wives and children behind and are celebrated for their accomplishments? How many centuries did women live in the shadow of their men? I love being a mother, I love being a wife, but it is not in my nature to be submissive in this role. I am a woman, a person of my own dreams and desires. It is something I wanted to show by example to my daughters and to my son. If you want to love me, you have to take me for who I am. Often that will not be an easy task. The children possess unconditional love, but men who are attracted to women of strong and independent character often don't quite know how to let go of them when they need to fly free for a while and trust they will return. In trust lies the deepest form of love.

I comforted myself that my son, Tilen, was coming in two days. We would have a special alone time, just the two of us. We didn't get to do that very often anymore.

I climbed the last hill out of the arroyo and cresting the top, I turned through the wide-open, black iron gate into my driveway. My friend and her daughter had left it open for me. Just like that, I was *home*. I stood there leaning on the bike, waiting for a deluge of tears, but none came. Pressing my hands against my eyes, I could smell the miles embedded in my mold-covered gloves. There I was, standing alone in the home I'd been longing to reach, holding onto an idea that was solemnly mine.

I had arrived at a place I so desperately wanted to call home. But no place is a home without your people. I had expectations. I wanted my man and my dog to be there to greet me. Expectations are just empty promises we give ourselves, causing pain when they're not met. An endless learning process for me. I'd made my own choices, and I was living with them. No, I was living *them*.

I still sought Jim's approval. I wanted him to be proud of me, of what I'd accomplished. I was that little girl again, seeking approval from my father.

I put the bike into storage, set the mattress on our outdoor concrete bed, and set up the outdoor kitchen. I went to take a much-needed shower, and I found myself surrounded by so many dear and familiar things. Shampoo, a whole bar of soap, a sharp razor with which I could finally shave my legs and armpits for the first time in nearly two months. My legs resembled those of a woolly mammoth. All that hair, which had been nonexistent during my chemo treatments, had returned with a vengeance. I'd never been so thin, gaunt really. My body looked like a dried prune. All the muscle and whatever fat I'd had or was sensitive about having had melted away. I could without hesitation tell you that if you struggle with a few extra stubborn pounds, keep them. They make you look beautiful! At my age, being this thin just made me look older. My face stared back at me from the mirror, and etched in it was a roadmap of wrinkles resembling the dry, cracked desert I'd crossed. My left breast and whatever was left of my right one sagged sadly like turned-out pockets of an old, worn-out pair of jeans. They didn't look like they belonged to me. I didn't recognize the person staring back at me.

With a deep sigh, I opened a box of old clothes I kept at the house. A clean but stale-smelling shirt and underwear, and even an old bra, now a couple of sizes too large. Everything was such a luxury. I found an old but crispy clean pair of white cutoff jeans. I hadn't been able to wear them for years because they were too tight. I found no belt.

Everything was falling off me. I cut up my old sarong and fashioned a belt out of it to hold up my shorts.

I headed out to meet Jerry and his family at Las Palmas restaurant. As his kids climbed into my lap, my stomach still struggled to keep food down. I ordered a cup of chamomile tea. I was happy but physically and emotionally exhausted.

The trip soon caught up with me. I said goodnight to a jolly group of friends and drove home. I fell into my bed under the open palapa. I was gone. It was the first night in a very, very long time that nothing woke me.

At dawn, I heard a bird. It is always one bird first, like the conductor of a symphonic orchestra raising his hand to indicate that music is about to start and everyone in the orchestra needs to get their instruments at attention. After that first chirp, the music started. I lay there in the red glow of the early morning. I was warm under my down comforter. My head rested on a soft down pillow. The Sea of Cortez appeared oily and inky black. A slight morning mist sat on the horizon, helping the blood-orange sky change to apricot sorbet and rusty caramel. Plenty of time still before the sea gave birth to a giant red ball of fire. I closed my eyes and allowed myself to drift back to sleep. I felt so safe. I had no place I had to go!

Appropriately, it was Thanksgiving Day, and I had so much to be thankful for. My whole life was captured there, at that very moment. I have never felt more content, more at peace than at that moment, lying in my bed, in the safety of my own home. I had journeyed so far. I was tired but, on that morning, for the first time, tired felt good.

—TWENTY-EIGHT—
The Feast of All Feasts

You go away for a long time and return a different person—
you never come all the way back.
—Paul Theroux

I went to the doctor in town to get checked. I stepped on the scale, and it showed forty-four kilograms, which was ninety-seven pounds, the weight with which I entered high school and was still growing. The doctor prescribed antibiotics. My skin was paper-thin and dry. I could hardly squeeze any urine out for the test, and it was dark yellow, almost orange and cloudy. The doctor sent me home with three liters of electrolytes and asked me to return the next day for a follow-up test. She was very concerned about my kidneys. Any further dehydration could cause the whole system to fail. I was worried, as I'd had serious issues with my kidneys as a child. I'd spent my entire third grade in the hospital after kidney surgeries.

I was invited to Thanksgiving dinner at a friend's house. As I entered their beautiful home, the tables were loaded with platters of food. It was the feast of all Thanksgiving feasts. The aroma of a golden-brown turkey reached me way before I entered the house. My senses had sharpened by several degrees during my ride. Everyone was in a festive mood. It felt so good to be surrounded by people I knew.

"Well, we all sure are glad you made it!" Joel said, giving me a big bear hug.

"We were all so worried about you!" Shelly said. "I had Glen ready to go get you at a moment's notice." She looked at her husband. "We were all watching your progress. We were all so worried about you!"

I didn't realize how many people had followed my trip. I felt so much love! I nibbled on appetizers. Everything felt so normal. But I was also not used to being surrounded by so many people. After being on my own for so long, it was all quite overwhelming, and I struggled for words.

At dinnertime, I loaded my plate, and there was a rainbow of green peas, orange squash, red beets, white potatoes, and hardly any space left for a slice of delicious turkey with crispy skin dripping with fat and juices. I took five hurried bites, hardly making a dent on my plate, and I was full. Such gluttony, especially now after my two-month-long ride, where food was such a scarce luxury. I took a sip of wine. I love wine, but it didn't taste right to me. I excused myself and headed to the bathroom. The food and the wine had made me sick. I felt guilty I couldn't eat all that lovingly prepared, sumptuous, glorious food. I caught a glance of myself in the mirror. I saw a dried-up pumpkin in an orange blouse looking back at me. My hair still felt and looked like straw, even though I'd washed it with regular shampoo and conditioner. Funny! I didn't have to think about how I looked when I was riding all by myself.

Two days later, I was running around in anticipation, getting the place ready for Tilen's arrival. I looked forward to enjoying time riding our bikes, and if the wind gods were favorable, we would go kitesurfing together. I was excited out of my mind. I was in the upstairs room we'd built for the kids when they were little. It was a simple room, brim full of memories. I had cleaned and was making the bed when the shuttle arrived from San Jose del Cabo airport. I ran downstairs to greet Tilen. I saw a bearded man walking toward me and somewhere in that beard was a huge grin, his eyes sparkling with joy and love. My twenty-three-year-old mountain man was here. We hugged but then, from behind the red suburban jumped Jana.

"Surprise!" she shrieked.

"Oh, my god! Jana!" I screamed. I cried and cried, and then we all hugged and danced in a circle. "You little shit!" I yelled joyfully at my daughter, who was happily grinning in my direction.

"Mom!" said Tilen. "You're so skinny! We're going to have to put some meat back on those bones!" he said, laughing, but I heard concern in his voice.

"So, where are we going tonight to celebrate?" asked Jana.

"Let's start at Baja Joes, and we'll take it from there," I said. "Go clean up. We have plenty of time. I wish Mateja was here."

"We tried to get her to come, Mom. She really wanted to, but she couldn't take time off from work. She wishes she was here!"

"I know, I know. She's with us here."

It was impossible to describe the joy I felt hugging my children.

"How about a mountain bike ride, Mom?" asked Tilen. "Have you ridden your bike yet since you got here?"

"Nope," I said. "I haven't even unloaded it yet. The Beast is resting. I am resting. Tomorrow morning though. We'll all go for a ride tomorrow morning."

In the morning, I finally unloaded and cleaned The Beast. We rode on single-track trails behind our house. Without all the extra weight, the bike felt jittery, and it took me a while to get used to it. As I rode, I said to Tilen and Jana, "The Beast served me well. Only one flat tire the whole way. I owe Wayne at the Olympic bike shop a six-pack of beer."

I never would have believed it was possible not to have any real issues with the bike on such a long and rough journey. I think big tall Wayne is going to be happy to hear that.

We rode, we swam, we ate. My stomach was finally feeling better, and when I returned to the doctor in town, my kidneys had stabilized. However, she told me to continue drinking plenty of water and electrolytes. I was slowly regaining my strength and was happy to be with my kids. It all felt so easy, normal, and happy.

Then they left, Jana after three short days, and then Tilen a day later. They both had to go back to work. I was alone again, waiting for Jim. He finally departed from Tahoe with our friend Paul. I anticipated their arrival in about three days if all went well.

It came down to a few more hours of waiting. I got the place cleaned and ready for them. I was nervous and all worked up in anticipation. Two months doesn't seem like a long time, but to me, at that moment, it was an eternity. So much had happened to me, with me. It felt like a lifetime. How we think about time is such a strange thing. Einstein said, "The faster you move, the slower the time moves." For nearly two months, I had been in constant motion. I'd perceived that time differently than someone who had been relatively stationary in one place. I'd gone through a metamorphosis. I was worried, though. How did Jim feel? He had been through so much stress worrying about me. He worked so hard and struggled with his own medical issues, and I was not there to care for him. Was he angry with me? I felt a high level of guilt.

Years ago, my friend Scott had said to me, "Alenka, you worry too much! You have both kinds of guilt."

"Oh? What do you mean?" I asked.

"Well," he explained, "your Catholic guilt for everything that happened in the past, and your Jewish guilt for everything which will happen in the future!"

My friend Laraine called me, and we went paddleboarding. Moving across the water and talking to my dear friend was a good distraction. But it didn't last long.

"I have to go back, Laraine. I need to be home when Jim arrives," I said nervously.

I ran home and jumped in the shower. I wanted to look good. I wanted to look fresh for Jim.

I came out of the shower, and as I was walking toward the storage room where we kept our clothes, wrapped in a towel, still dripping wet, my hair a mess, Jim came around the corner. Monty came running from behind him, and when he saw me, crouched down for a second and then started running circles around me as if he were possessed. He finally stopped and lay down on his back at my feet. In all his excitement, he peed on himself. Jim and I stood a few feet apart with Monty between us, and we were motionless, staring at each other, not knowing what to do. It was the most awkward moment.

"Are you mad at me, Jim?" I asked quietly,

"No, of course not. Why would I be mad at you?"

"I think Monty is a bit more excited to see me than you are." I knew he heard the hurt in my voice.

Paul was standing in the middle of our palapa, behind us, watching the scene.

"Are you going to hug your wife or what, man?"

Jim finally whispered in my ear.

"You are one crazy woman, but I'm glad you are mine." He leaned in and added, "It was just . . . it was just that you were gone too long."

It was halting, but it was also beautiful to hear.

Finally, the distance between us disappeared, and I melted into Jim. The time between our last embrace in Yosemite, almost two months earlier, faded away as we hugged. I just needed to be held, and I couldn't feel the ground beneath me.

—TWENTY-NINE—
The Mountains Crashing
into the Sea

*When I come back home from a trip, one of the first things I
need to do is walk into my kitchen and look around. It always
makes me feel better, when I know exactly where I am.*
—Alice Waters

I knew I needed to go back and finish riding the missing link I'd
skipped when I got sick. For nearly two months, the thought of that
unfinished business kept me awake at night. One of the first things
my son asked me when he arrived to La Ventana from the airport was,
"So, Mom, when are you going to go back to finish the ride between
Constitucion and La Paz?"

I knew he was right, though I wasn't ready for that question yet.
But how could I disappoint my own son?

The trip was only three days long, but every time I packed and got
ready to go, something came up, and then I would feel relieved to
have an excuse not to go. I was even happy when I came down with
a case of bronchitis for the whole month of January. How difficult it
was to leave the comfort and safety of my home again!

I dreaded the thought of leaving Jim. We were slowly getting
used to each other again, but there was tension between us as well.

Whenever I brought it up, he didn't want to talk about my going back to finish the ride. I hated the thought of leaving him alone to worry about me again, especially after a young hiker went missing in the nearby mountains. Police, army, and organized private searches went on day and night. With every day that went by, the chances of finding him alive faded. There was no trace of him, and to this day, his body has not been found. Apprehension hung in the air like woodsmoke. I was hesitant to tempt my fate again. What if I'd just been lucky?

Yet, every time I walked by the bike and the box with my gear neatly packed, I felt The Beast calling me back. "We've come too far. We're not done."

I've had a particular experience of unfinished business in my past.

The spring of my freshman year in college, I went on a backcountry ski trip to Mount Jalovec, one of the Julian Alps ski touring classics. The highlight of skiing that majestic, sharp-edged, rocky, pyramid-shaped mountain was a steep couloir leading to the summit. A blizzard raged that day, and it was cold, but that meant the snow was light. My boyfriend, Andrej, his climbing partner, and I were making our way up the mountain. They had been backcountry skiing for years and had all the proper gear. Since I was a ski racer, I only had racing equipment. My boots had a very tight fit, with no extra room to wiggle my toes to help circulation, so my feet froze. I was miserable. I was walking up the mountain, carrying my racing skis strapped to my backpack, and in deep snow I sank up to my knees. In drifts created by strong winds, I would sink all the way to my waist. I was also terrified of the high avalanche danger. That mountain is known for avalanches killing people. I fell behind the boys.

"You guys go ahead. I'll catch up with you!" I yelled after them, my voice swallowed by the fog, wind, and snow.

The two silhouettes moved farther up the mountain and soon

disappeared. I found shelter behind a big boulder and waited, freezing my ass off. Minutes stretched into an hour, then two. I was shivering and cursing myself for giving up too soon. By the time I changed my mind, it was too late to follow. I dozed off and woke up to voices calling my name, emerging from the fog and the curtain of the falling snow. They were the voices of sheer exuberance. I stood up from my shelter to meet my friends. "Oh you won't believe how great the snow was in the couloir. Best powder ever. Perfect pitch. Best turns of our life," Andrej and his friend boasted.

I hated them both, but I hated myself more. We headed back down to the valley and caught the last bus home. I didn't say a word the whole way home. I brooded the entire week during classes. I had to go back. The next Saturday, I talked my dad into going to ski Mount Jalovec again. This time we were able to drive a car into Planica Valley and all the way to Tamar hut, so our approach to the base of the mountain was much shorter. The conditions were miserable. It was springtime, and the snow that had fallen the previous weekend had turned to mush. The debris from several avalanches crossed our path.

"Good thing you weren't caught in this last weekend," my dad said, with much concern in his voice.

He begged me to turn around and ski back down.

"We can come back," he said. "This snow is terrible, and it isn't safe."

For the umpteenth time, he fell to his waist through rotten snow covering low brush, muttering, *Ti prekleta trmasta koza!*

I understood the words all too well. Once again, I'd had been called a damn stubborn goat.

We were post-holing, sinking deep with nearly every step we took. My dad stopped at my boulder.

"I think I'll just wait here for you. I get it. You need to go to the top. I don't."

He understood I wasn't going to quit this time.

By sheer grit, stupidity, and determination, I made it to the top of the couloir, reached Kotovo saddle, and clicked into my bindings. The skiing down was complete crap. Sticky snow made turning difficult, so I had to use a hop-and-turn technique all the way through deep, mushy snow that wanted to swallow me every time I landed a turn. Once I reconnected with my dad, I was worried about him, and I knew that if anything had happened to him, it would have been my fault. I could hear him cursing behind me all the way to the car. Every third word was *koza* and truly feeling guilty to be that stubborn goat, I was afraid to turn around and see him crashing over and over.

When we reached the car, my dad sat down in the passenger seat and handed me the keys, something he normally wouldn't do.

"You drive!"

He leaned his head back and immediately started snoring. Throughout my life, this Jalovec tour served as a reminder of how much unfinished business eats at me.

On January 2, 2019, I turned fifty-five. What a cool number! Half a century with half a decade tacked on. Now, there was something to celebrate! I loved being fifty-five! "Fifty-five, fifty-five!" I could say it out loud without it sounding strange or scary to me. I had fulfilled my dream, I'd stood on my own two feet, I felt strong and proud I'd accomplished something greater than myself. Age just didn't seem that important any longer.

We built a giant bonfire on the beach with friends and howled at the full moon late into the night. I walked away from the jolly group and went to sit on a log that had washed up at the edge of the water. Gentle waves lapped the shore, and as I dipped my toes into the ocean, they looked as if they were covered with blue glitter. They glowed bright, bathed by bioluminescent plankton. I watched people dancing and singing around the fire from a distance in the darkness. The persistent, nagging thought was still tugging at my heart: *Your journey isn't finished*!

Finally, an opportunity arrived in February. I met up with young Hannah, a niece of friends of ours from Tahoe. She was approaching Ciudad Constitution, riding her bike down the Baja Divide. Her plan was to meet with her uncle and her father to ride my missing section of the divide, but storms had delayed her dad and uncle. Instead of them, I met up with this twenty-two-year-old Amazonian warrior. It was a good compromise for Jim. He was more relaxed because I had someone to ride with.

Hannah and I started in the rain on the morning of February 6. Smoke and mist rose from the dump on the outskirts of the city where Jim dropped us off.

"See you in three days, girls!" he yelled, watching us ride away while Monty chased after cows rummaging through the trash. As I turned to wave one last goodbye, Jim was slumped over, just like he had been every time they wheeled me off into one of my many surgeries over the past three years.

Hannah kicked my ass right out of the gate. No way could I keep up with her! I realized my mistake in the first few miles, chasing after her. We rode in suffocating humidity on a long, flat, and unremarkable section of a sandy washboard road that led us toward Mission Gonzaga. From there, we finally entered a more interesting canyon land. The road started climbing. I pushed as hard as I could but fell behind. My damaged leg was cramping like never before. I screamed in pain, feeling completely disconnected from my first trip, wishing

I'd gone by myself. I wouldn't have felt the pressure to keep up. It was beautiful, though, and we rode through stunning canyons, passing remote mountain villages, riding by many ranchos. Just like it had been on the rest of my trip through Baja, people were incredibly friendly.

"Que le vaya bien!" May it go well! Kids were yelling and waving as we rode past their school.

Hannah is an old soul. It was beautiful camping on a high plateau among the cacti the first night. We built Hannah's first fire of her trip and watched the stars until clouds moved in and the rain chased us into our tents. On the second day, we climbed over steep, rocky roads over the final pass, and the mountains crashed back into the Sea of Cortez. I knew of a small sandy cove, and there we spent our second night, sitting by the fire with bright Venus, Jupiter, and Mars lined up for our viewing. It was nice to have conversations and marvel over the beautiful sunset colors. The north winds howled the whole night, five-foot waves crashing onto the beach. The tent flysheet was flapping all night loudly, not allowing for much sleep.

We packed up early, well before sunrise when the sky showed off a spectacular palette of reds and oranges. I was eager to start riding early. We had a long day ahead and had to cover over a hundred miles to reach La Paz.

We rode off at dawn and were greeted immediately by a steep punishing climb. The last part of the ride toward La Paz led us along mountains eroded by water, wind and sun, creating flat top colorful landforms called mesas. They looked like giant, layered, multicolored wedding cakes. The Sea of Cortez was to our left. We were on our home stretch, and I was counting kilometer markers on the side of the road one by one, praying for the ride to be over.

In the distance, I saw a van, I saw a man, and I saw a dog sitting next to the man. They shimmered like a mirage on the side of the road in the heat rising from the pavement. It was a scene I had envisioned so many times on my ride down Baja Peninsula. I breathed a big sigh of relief and fulfillment as if I'd just reached the top of a mountain I'd wanted to climb all my life. I realized that my trip was now truly complete. There was the man I had chosen, waiting for me with our beautiful dog, Monty, by his side!

Epilogue

Starting in Tahoe, riding up and down the spine of Upper and Lower California mountains until I reached La Ventana Bay, I had climbed 158,263 feet or 48,238 vertical meters, which is like scaling Mount Everest from sea level to summit nearly five and a half times. I covered 2,524 miles or 4,062 kilometers in fifty-seven days. People asked me all the time, "How many miles did you ride?" Or "How long did it take you?" Do these statistics matter? Sure they do, but only because every mile was a part of my physical and inner journey. With every rotation of the wheels, The Beast took me up and down the mountains into the wind, through freezing temperatures in the Sierra Nevada Mountains, crossing scorching hot and barren desert plains, over rough, remote rocky roads, through deep soft sand, across the salt flats along the Pacific, revealed something new and different inside of me. It opened deeply buried wounds, made them raw again before they were scabbed over, and also made them a bit less obvious, a bit more bearable. Every laborious breath I took told me I was doing this because I wanted to, not because I was forced to do it by circumstances out of my control. It was difficult, but I chose this less-traveled road.

So, yes, one road diverged in the woods and was less traveled.

But it was my road because this is who I am, this is who I have always been, this is who I will always be. Still searching for the path to my true self. Always moving forward, never giving up.

Before I took this trip, I didn't think of it as a pilgrimage. What is a pilgrimage? Phil Cousineau describes it in his book, *The Art of Pilgrimage:* "Pilgrimage means following the footsteps of somebody or something we honor to pay homage. It revitalizes our lives, reinvigorates our very souls."

But what was my pilgrimage? If I have ever worshiped and admired anyone or wanted to follow the path of anyone else in my life, it is the mountain climbers, adventure seekers, and misfits on a quest to discover new, impossible things, searching for the deeper meaning in life. I felt the gravitational pull I couldn't—or better yet, didn't want to—resist. My journey on The Beast was my Mount Everest, the dream of a fourteen-year-old girl. And why did I dream of Everest? Because the mountain is so massive it affects the gravity around it. The gravity that pulls us toward something impossible, something we need to conquer.

Once the idea of the ride entered my brain, it lodged itself there, like a stubborn pebble in your shoe which must be removed. Perhaps I didn't even understand why the pull to go on this journey was so strong. Somewhere along the way, the healing process of my body and my soul began. The journey, especially riding through Mexico, which has always been a sacred place for me, was irrevocably transformative. Even though I had a goal to ride from my home in Lake Tahoe, California to my home in La Ventana Bay, Mexico, what I found was my *way* by living the life I was born to live. I listened to the advice of mountaineer Nejc Zaplotnik: "He who is in pursuit of a goal will remain empty once he has attained it. But he who has found the way, will always carry the goal with him."

I was always the person beating my own drum, I only wanted to awaken my own dying spirit, stoke the extinguished fire within, and follow through on dreams I'd conceived all those years ago. I wasn't running away from anyone, except that I was seriously sick of all the doctors, endless testing, medications, and uncertainties. I wanted to accomplish something bigger than myself, while I still had the time and ability to do it.

Somewhere along the way, sitting alone in the desert under the vast sky littered with stars and planets and galaxies beyond, I started to feel a shift inside. I began to feel the lightness and confidence I'd been searching for. I reached the point of no return.

On my pilgrimage, I was swallowed by the rhythm of the pedals ascending and descending from dawn to dusk and beyond.

The wind in my newly grown hair eased my concerns about an end nearing swiftly and too soon.

The sweat that dripped between my one and a half breasts and dried into a salty crust on my weathered skin allowed my faith in things good to return.

People I met along the way who had the least gave me the most.

I was surrounded by space devoid of people, noise, and material overabundance, and I screamed with newfound joy into the air around me when no one could hear me. I experienced a feeling I could call pure bliss, nirvana, or whatever you want to name the balancing of internal and external forces—those same forces that, before my journey, pulled me apart.

Fears I faced and fought.

I was touched by ancient spirits that guided and protected me on the fringes of loneliness.

I crossed the deserts while the Mexican sun sucked the last ounce of fluids from my prune-like body, until faith was restored again by gulping down sweet water handed to me by a stranger.

It wasn't until I sat on the porch with a vaquero in the remote mountains, his wide-brimmed hat shading his gazing eyes, who, with a sweeping motion of his gnarled hand, showed me my way back home. It was then that I recognized the shape of my journey.

In the end, I did find my home. Just like the journey itself, home is a state of mind. It lives in our soul and our heart. It is what we create with the people we love, and we take it everywhere we go. It was all there before I left. My family, my home, and my faithful golden retriever, Monty. But I had to go out on two wheels and find out for myself, and as it was my luck, I left the doors ajar just enough to enable me to return to the safety and embrace of the man who, in the end, was strong enough to allow me to be myself. He allowed me to follow my dreams, which were conceived on the banks of the river in the shade of the mountains in the home I left so long ago.

Is my search complete? Not until the day breath leaves my body, and I return to this earth as a golden retriever chasing tennis balls, making someone else happy.

Acknowledgments

There are no shortcuts to writing a book. I am deeply humbled and grateful for the help of so many people who encouraged me along the way, especially my family. I thank you for all the love, support, and understanding during the past few years, when all I could do and think of was writing this book. Not an easy task for someone whose native language isn't English. Most of all, thank you, Jim Granger, my husband and the love of my life, for bringing me coffee in bed in the wee hours of the morning, so I could write when my mind was still fresh. I am so grateful to you for your unwavering love and support.

In March 2018, I attended a weeklong yoga retreat in Baja, California, with Jenni Fox and Paul Gould. At the end of the week, we were all asked to write our intentions. The words I put down on paper, *I will write a book*, changed my life. The need to sever the marriage portion of my relationship to the father of my three children and slip silently out of the darkness toward the light, hoping to find my own path, my own center, was where I started. I wrote one paragraph. I realized I needed something else to tie together all the events of my life.

At the end of that same spring, our friends Blake and Maggie Bockius came to Baja to ride bikes on the Cape Loop section of Baja Divide. It was the first time I'd heard about the seventeen-hundred-mile-long Baja Divide Bikepacking Route. Starting at the California–Mexico border, it connects the Pacific Ocean and the Sea of Cortez, crossing every major mountain range in Baja California and ending in La Paz, only thirty-five miles from my second home. Listening to Blake's descriptions of the challenges and dangers of the ride made me question the sanity of anyone even attempting to ride a bike through such a hostile yet unmistakably fascinating environment. Somehow, the idea of riding from my home in Tahoe through the mountains of California to my second home in Baja lodged in my mind, and I couldn't get rid of it. Wasn't that my dream? Didn't I write it fifteen years earlier in my Rumi pocketbook? I always wanted to accomplish one thing larger than myself before I disappeared into the shadows of time. My time was running out, so in the end of September of that year, I left my home in Lake Tahoe, California, on a fully loaded bike I called The Beast, having no clue what I was getting myself into. Call it gutsy or stupid, maybe both, as I had never bike-packed in my life. I wrote the blog along the way, and with the help of my daughter Mateja, posted it on the web for my family and friends. People I didn't even know followed the blog. They encouraged me not just to continue my difficult journey, but also to write a book. I am so grateful to you all, especially Mateja. Without her, the blog, and probably the book, wouldn't have materialized.

In March 2019, after I completed the bike ride, my dear friends Marilyn Crang and Mary Ann Milford told me I should attend the annual Travel Writers Conference organized by Book Passage Book Store in Corte Madera. The conference was a life-changing experience. The most challenging journey of my life—writing the book—began.

Don George taught me that travel writing should always be about the meaning of life. Phil Cousineau believed in my story and saw that I was coachable. He spent endless hours reading my first disheveled manuscript draft and helped me look for the story within the story. Whenever I felt like giving up, I'd receive a postcard from Phil, encouraging me to keep on writing. I thank you Phil, for teaching me the Art of Pilgrimage.

At the Book Passage Conference, I attended a three-day writing workshop with Larry Habbeger. In that class, the story of my beekeeper grandfather was born, and it unearthed memories of the sights, smells, textures, tastes, and sounds from my childhood. During our meetings in the cafes of San Francisco, I came to understand and appreciate the hard work and knowledge of book editors who have patience to put up with a lot of—let me just put it plainly—crappy writing. Thank you, Larry. I wrote and rewrote the manuscript so many times I lost count, but I was learning. I was growing, and what a gift that is at any age. Lockdown because of COVID came at the best possible time for me. I had no excuse to do anything but eat, drink, sleep and breathe writing. Attending online writing workshops with incredible teachers like Sands Hall, Don George, Judyth Hill, Janet Fitch, Peter Orner, and others from the comfort of my home was invaluable. Thank you, Suzanne Roberts, for introducing me to Kathryn (Kate) Miles. Kate took time to help me amid writing her own book, *Trailed*. Her mentorship was invaluable. She tore the manuscript apart and started moving the pieces of the story like a giant puzzle, giving it a more coherent flow, additional depth. Thank you, Kate. I am forever grateful.

On our weekly group bike rides in Baja, I learned that Mark Larabee was an author, a Pulitzer Prize-winning journalist, and an editor. It took me a while to find the courage to ask if he would read my manuscript. He kindly agreed. I told him not to be nice to the manuscript just because he knew me. Together, we continued to explore ways in and around sensitive subjects. I tended to skip or speed through the most painful and shameful parts of my life, as I didn't want to drag people through the mud or hurt anyone. Mistakes were made on all sides. Mark, along with my other incredible editors, helped me (I sincerely hope) to tell my story with grace. Mark had another challenge while combing through my manuscript: He had to delete hundreds of occurrences of *actually*. I didn't realize how often I used that word until Mark (actually) pointed it out to me. Mark, you are a dear friend, and I look forward to many more debates drinking tequila and eating great food in our special corner of the world.

Professor Tom Spradley helped me navigate the Baja night sky and made sure that all the correct planets and stars were aligned. I hope they name one of the newborn stars discovered by the James Webb telescope after Tom and his lovely wife Louise.

There are more friends like Tim Hauserman, Laura Read, Carol Hanner, and countless others I know I need to thank. It truly takes a village to give birth to a book. By sharing my own journey, which has often been painful, I hope I can shed some light on the sufferings and strength of others.

About the Author

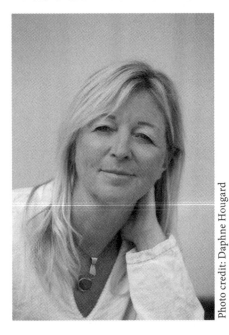

Photo credit: Daphne Hougard

A lenka Vrecek was born at the foot of the Alps in Slovenia, a part of former communist Yugoslavia. Born with a spirit for adventure, she came to America at twenty years old with a backpack, a pair of skis, and a pocket full of dreams. She was a ski coach and a director of Pedagogy for Squaw Valley and Alpine Meadows Ski Teams for thirty years. Alenka owns Tahoe Tea Company and lives in Lake Tahoe, California, with her second husband, Jim, their four children, three grandchildren, and a Golden Retriever named Monty.

SELECTED TITLES FROM SHE WRITES PRESS

She Writes Press is an independent publishing company founded to serve women writers everywhere. Visit us at www.shewritespress.com.

Brave(ish): A Memoir of a Recovering Perfectionist by Margaret Davis Ghielmetti. $16.95, 978-1-63152-747-0

An intrepid traveler sets off at forty to live the expatriate dream over-seas—only to discover that she has no idea how to live even her own life. Part travelogue and part transformation tale, Ghielmetti's memoir, narrated with humor and warmth, proves that it's never too late to reconnect with our authentic selves—if we dare to put our own lives first at last.

Bowing to Elephants: Tales of a Travel Junkie by Mag Dimond
$16.95, 978-1-63152-596-4

Mag Dimond, an unloved girl from San Francisco, becomes a travel junkie to avoid the fate of her narcissistic, alcoholic mother—but every-where she goes, she's haunted by memories of her mother's neglect, and by a hunger to find out who she is, until she finds peace and her authentic self in the refuge of Buddhist practice.

She Rode a Harley: A Memoir of Love and Motorcycles by Mary Jane Black. $16.95, 978-1-63152-620-6

After escaping an abusive marriage, Mary Jane finds love with Dwayne, who teaches her to ride a Harley; traveling together, they learn to be partners, both on and off the road, until Dwayne gets cancer. Without him, Mary Jane once again must learn to live on her own—but she'll never be the same again.

Blue Apple Switchback: A Memoir by Carrie Highley
$16.95, 978-1-63152-037-2

At age forty, Carrie Highley finally decided to take on the biggest switch-back of her life: upon her bicycle, and with the help of her mentor's wisdom, she shed everything she was taught to believe as a young lady growing up in the South—and made a choice to be true to herself and everyone else around her.